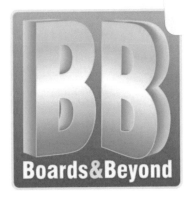

Boards and Beyond:
Neurology

A Companion Book to the Boards and Beyond Website

Jason Ryan, MD, MPH

2018 Edition

Table of Contents

Cells of the Nervous System

Jason Ryan, MD, MPH

Nervous System Cells

- Neurons
- Astrocytes
- Microglia
- Oligodendroglia
- Schwann cells

Glial Cells

- Support neurons
- Macroglia
  - Astrocytes, oligodendrocytes, ependyma
- Microglia
- Gliosis:
  - Proliferation/hypertrophy of glial cells
  - Reaction to CNS injury
  - Astrocytes undergo major changes
- Glioma
  - Astrocytoma, Oligodendroglioma, Ependymomas

Neurons

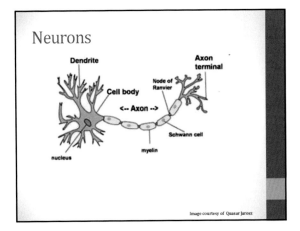

Image courtesy of Quasar Jarosz

Neuron Action Potentials
Key Facts

- At rest, neurons have voltage of -70mV
- This is maintained by "leak" of K+ out of cell
- To depolarize, Na channels open
- This allows Na into cell and raises voltage
- Na channels open along axon → propagation
- At axon terminal, Ca channels open
- Triggers release of neurotransmitter
- Vesicles fuse with membrane → exocytosis

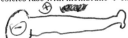

Action Potential

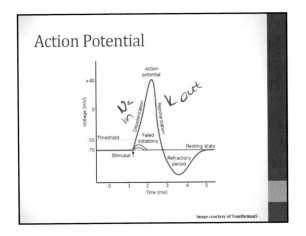

Image courtesy of Tomtheman5

Clinical Relevance

- Agents that block Na channels will inhibit signals
- Local anesthetics
  - Lidocaine, Benzocaine, Tetracaine, Cocaine, etc.
- Some neurotoxins block Na channels
  - Pufferfish → tetrodotoxin
  - Japanese food

Astrocytes

- Important for support of neurons
- Found in CNS: Gray and white matter
- Removes excess neurotransmitter
- Repair, scar formation
- Major part of reactive gliosis
  - Hypertrophy
  - Hyperplasia
- GFAP is key astrocyte marker

Astrocytes
Clinical Relevance

- Astrocytomas
  - Cerebellum of children
  - GFAP positive
- JC Virus infects astrocytes and oligodendrocytes
  - Causes PML in HIV patients

Microglia

- CNS macrophages
- Proliferate in response to injury
- Differentiate into larger phagocytes after injury
- HIV can persist in the brain via microglia
- Chronic HIV encephalitis: nodules of activated microglia

Oligodendroglia

- Myelinate CNS axons
- Each cell myelinates multiple axons
- Most common glial cell in white matter
- Destroyed in multiple sclerosis

Schwann Cells

- Myelinate PNS axons
- Each cell myelinates one axons
- Very important for neuron regeneration
- Destroyed in Guillain-Barre syndrome
- Form Schwannomas
  - Also called acoustic neuromas
  - Classically affect CN VIII

Myelin

- Lipids and proteins
- Increases SPEED of impulse propagation in axon
- Saltatory Conduction
  - Only need to depolarize Nodes of Ranvier
  - Do not need to depolarize entire axon
  - This makes process faster
  - ↑ conduction velocity
  - ↑ length constant
- CNS: Oligodendrocytes
- PNS: Schwann cells

decay to ⅓
of original potential

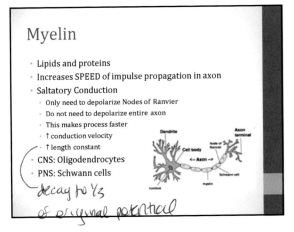

Types of Nerve Fibers

- Classification by diameter, myelin
- A-alpha:
  - Large, myelinated fibers, 6 to 15 microns diameter
  - Most efferent motor fibers
  - Touch, vibration, and position
- A-delta
  - Small, myelinated fibers, 3 to 5 microns in diameter
  - Cold, pain
- C fibers
  - Unmyelinated fibers, 0.5 to 2 microns in diameter
  - Warm, pain

Large

Small

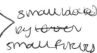
small dia by small fibers

How Nerves Sense

- Four structures on nerve ending allow us to sense the world
- Free nerve endings
- Meissner's Corpuscles
- Pacinian Corpuscles
- Merkel's disks

Free Nerve Endings

- Mostly found in skin
- Sense pain and temperature
- Separate pain, cold and warm receptors
- C and A-delta fibers

Meissner's Corpuscles

- Touch receptors
- Located near surface of skin
- Concentrated sensitive areas like fingers
  - "Glabrous" (hairless) skin
- Deformed by pressure → nerve stimulation
- A-alpha (large, myelinated) fibers

Pacinian Corpuscles

- Vibration, pressure receptors
- Located deep skin, joints, ligaments
- Egg-shaped structure
- Layers of tissue around free nerve ending
- Deformed by pressure → nerve stimulation
- A-alpha (large, myelinated) fibers

Merkel's Discs

- Pressure, position receptors
- Many locations, but especially hair follicles
- A-alpha (large, myelinated) fibers
- Sustained response to pressure
  - "Slowly adapting"
  - Provide continues information
- Contrast with Meissner's, Pacinian
  - "Rapidly adapting"
  - Respond mostly to *changes*

Peripheral Nerves

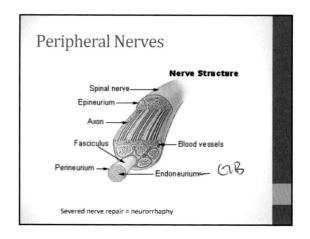

Severed nerve repair = neurorrhaphy

Nerve Damage

Jason Ryan, MD, MPH

Peripheral Nerve Damage

- Mild: Neurapraxia
- Moderate: Axonotmesis
- Severe: Neurotmesis
- Can result in weakness or sensory loss

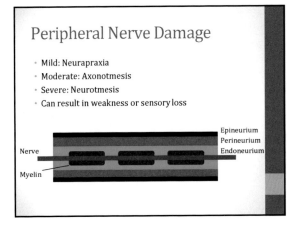

Neurapraxia

- Mild injury
- Focal demyelination
- Axon distal to injury intact
- Continuity across injury
- Excellent recovery

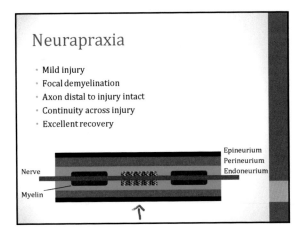

Neurotmesis

- Severe lesions
- Axon, myelin sheath irreversibly damaged
- External continuity of the injured nerve disrupted
- No significant regeneration occurs
- Bad prognosis

epi
peri
endo

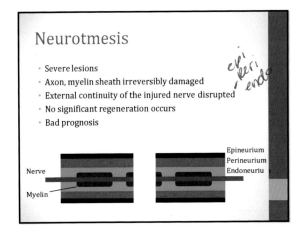

Axonotmesis

- Demyelination plus damage to axon
- Endoneurium, perineurium remain intact

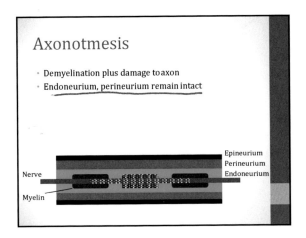

Axonotmesis

distal

- Distal to the lesion: "Wallerian degeneration"
  - Also occurs just proximal to injury
- Axon degenerates, myelin sheath involutes
- Axon regrowth sometimes occurs
- Possible if Schwann cells maintain integrity

Axonotmesis

- Proximal to the lesion: "**Axonal reaction**"
- Also called central chromatolysis
- Up-regulation of **protein synthesis** for repair
- Cell body changes
  - Swelling
  - **Chromatolysis** (disappearance of Nissl bodies)
  - Nucleus moves to periphery
- Resolves with time

Chromatolysis

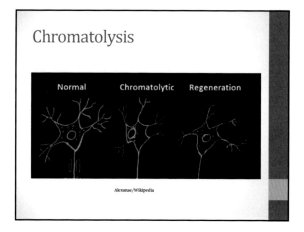

Alexanae/Wikipedia

Chromatolysis

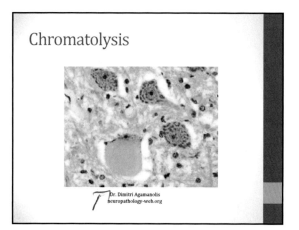

Dr. Dimitri Agamanolis
neuropathology-web.org

Axonotmesis

- Variable prognosis
  - Extent of damage
  - Distance to target
  - Complexity of nerve
- Usually partial recovery
- Longer recovery time than neurapraxia

Central Nerve Damage
Ischemia

- ~ 4-5 minutes of ischemia → irreversible damage
- **Neurons** more sensitive than glial cells
  - Higher energy demands; lack glycogen
- Most sensitive neurons:
  - Hippocampus
  - Purkinje cells (Cerebellum)
  - Neocortex
  - Striatum (Basal ganglia)

Central Nerve Damage
Changes after Infarction

- **12-24 hours**
  - No changes for about 12 hours
  - First changes occur in **neurons**
  - Microvacuoles (small holes) develop in neuron cytoplasm
  - Neurons become deep pink-red color "Red neurons"
  - Nucleus changes shape, color

Red Neurons

12-24 hours

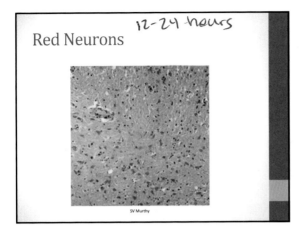

SV Murthy

Central Nerve Damage
Changes after Infarction

- **24-48 hours**
  - Neutrophils, macrophages, microglia
  - **Liquefactive necrosis from lysosomal enzymes release**

Central Nerve Damage
Changes after Infarction

- **Days to weeks**
  - Macrophages eliminate debris
  - Cyst forms
  - **Astrocytes undergo gliosis** - multiply, enlarge
  - Astrocyte processes form wall around cyst

UMN and LMN

- Somatics: two neuron chain
- Upper motor neuron
  - Brain to second nerve
- Lower motor neuron
  - CNS to muscle/target

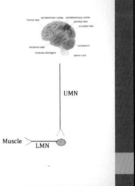

UMN

Muscle LMN

Image courtesy of Wikipedia and jkwchui

UMN and LMN

- UMN: Cortex, internal capsule, corticospinal tract
- LMN: Brainstem, spinal cord (anterior horn)

UMN and LMN

- Upper motor damage (pyramidal signs)
  - Spastic paralysis (stiff, rigid muscles)
  - Hyperreflexia
  - Muscle overactive
  - Clasp knife spasticity: passive movement → initial resistance, sudden release

UMN and LMN

- Lower motor damage
  - Flaccid paralysis
  - Fasciculation (spontaneous contractions/twitches)
  - Loss of reflexes

Decussation

- UMN cross just below medulla
  - Decussation
- Lesions above decussation
  - Contralateral dysfunction
- Lesions below decussation
  - Ipsilateral dysfunction

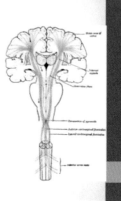

Bulbar

- Bulbar muscles are supplied by CN in brainstem
  - V (jaw)
  - VII (face)
  - IX (swallowing)
  - X (palate)
  - XI (head)
  - XII (tongue)

Bulbar vs. Pseudobulbar

- Bulbar palsy
  - Cranial nerve damage
  - LMN signs
- Pseudobulbar
  - Corticobulbar tract damage
  - UMN signs

Key Differences

- Bulbar
  - Absent jaw/gag reflex
  - Tongue flaccid/wasted
- Pseudobulbar
  - Exaggerated gag reflex
  - Tongue spastic (no wasting)
  - Spastic dysarthria

Blood Brain Barrier

Jason Ryan, MD, MPH

Blood Brain Barrier

- Surrounds CNS blood vessels
- Controls content CNS interstitial fluid
- Tight junctions btw endothelial cells of capillaries
- Astrocytes foot processes
  - Terminate in overlapping fashion on capillary walls

Blood Brain Barrier

- Water, some gases, and lipid soluble small molecules easily diffuse across
- Keeps out bacteria, many drugs
- Glucose/amino acids can't cross directly
  - Use carrier-mediated transport

Circumventricular Organs (CVO)

- Vascular brain structures around ventricles
- No blood brain barrier
- Allow communication CNS → blood stream
- Some sensory, some secretory
- Key CVOs
  - Area postrema
  - OVLT
  - Subfornical Organ (SFO)
  - Median Eminence of Hypothalamus

Area Postrema

- Caudal end of 4th ventricle in medulla
- "Chemoreceptor trigger zone"
- Outside blood brain barrier
- Chemo agents affect this area
- Sends signals to vomiting center in the medulla

OVLT

- Organum vasculosum of the lamina terminalis
- Anterior wall of the third ventricle
- Osmosensory neurons

Subfornical Organ (SFO)

- Anterior wall 3rd ventricle
- Responds to many circulating substances
- Exact roles not clear
- Responds to angiotensin II
- Projects to other brain areas

Median Eminence of Hypothalamus

- Releases hormones into vascular system to pituitary
- Allows hypothalamus to regulate pituitary

Other Brain Areas Without BBB

- Posterior Pituitary Gland
  - Oxytocin, ADH
- Pineal Gland
  - Melatonin

Vasogenic (Cerebral) Edema

- Breakdown of blood brain barrier
- Trauma, stroke
- Swelling of brain tissue

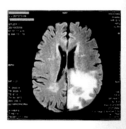

Image courtesy of Bobjgalindo

Neurotransmitters

Jason Ryan, MD, MPH

Peripheral Neurotransmitters

- Norepinephrine
- Acetylcholine
- Dopamine

Key CNS Neurotransmitters

- Norepinephrine ⎤ *PNS as well*
- Acetylcholine (ACh) ⎦
- Dopamine
- Serotonin (5-HT)
- γ-aminobutyric acid (GABA)
- Glutamate

Norepinephrine

- Stress/panic hormone
- Increased levels in anxiety
- Decreased levels in depression
  - Some antidepressants ↑NE levels
  - Serotonin–norepinephrine reuptake inhibitors (SNRIs)
  - Desipramine (TCA)
  - Monoamine Oxidase inhibitors (MAOi)

Locus Ceruleus

- Posterior pons near 4ᵗʰ ventricle
- Main source of NE in brain
- Critical for response to stress
- Extensive projections that activate under stress
- Activated in opiate withdrawal

Locus Ceruleus

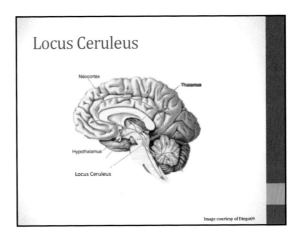

Image courtesy of Diego69

Dopamine

- Synthesized in:
  - Ventral tegmentum (midbrain)
  - Substantia nigra (midbrain)
- Increased levels in schizophrenia
- Decreased levels in Parkinson's
- Decreased levels in depression

Dopamine Synthesis

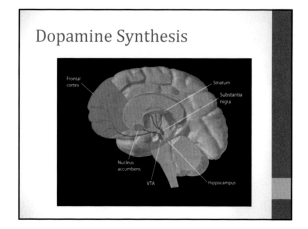

GABA

- γ-aminobutyric acid
- GABA is largely inhibitory
- Synthesized in nucleus accumbens (subcortex)
- Decreased levels in anxiety
- Decreased levels in Huntington's disease

GABA Synthesis

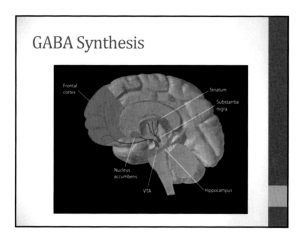

GABA Receptor Anesthetics

- Etomidate
- Propofol
- Benzodiazepines
- Barbiturates
- These drugs activate receptor → sedation

GABA Receptor

- GABA binds to receptor allows Cl⁻ into cell

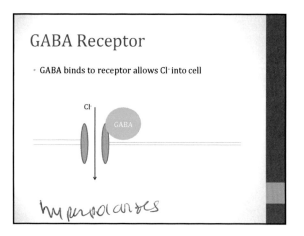

hyperpolarizes

GABA Synthesis

- Synthesized via glutamate decarboxylase in neurons
- Broken down by GABA transaminase
- Both enzymes need B6 cofactor

$\downarrow$ B6 = $\uparrow$ seizure

```
         Glutamate         GABA
        decarboxylase    Transaminase
Glutamate ──────────> GABA ──────────> Breakdown
                                         Products
```

GABA Receptor

- Three GABA receptor subtypes
- $GABA_A$ $GABA_B$ in brain
- $GABA_c$ in retina
- Benzodiazepines act on $GABA_A$
  - Stimulate Cl^- influx
- Alcohol, zolpidem, and barbiturates also $GABA_A$

Nucleus Accumbens

- Important for pleasure/reward
- Research shows NA activated in
  - Drug addiction
  - Fear

Serotonin

- Various functions
- Synthesized in raphe nucleus (pons)
- Decreased levels in anxiety
- Decreased levels in depression
  - Some antidepressants $\uparrow$5-HT levels
  - Selective-serotonin reuptake inhibitors (SSRIs)
  - Serotonin–norepinephrine reuptake inhibitors (SNRIs)
  - Monoamine Oxidase inhibitors (MAOi)

5-HT Synthesis

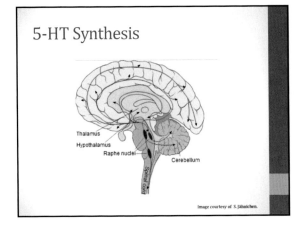

Image courtesy of S. Jähnichen.

Serotonin Syndrome

- Can occur any drug that that $\uparrow$serotonin
  - SSRIs, MAO inhibitors, SNRis, TCAs
- Classically triad
- #1: Mental status changes
  - Anxiety, delirium, restlessness, and disorientation
- #2: Autonomic hyperactivity
  - Diaphoresis, tachycardia, hyperthermia
- #3: Neuromuscular abnormalities
  - Tremor, clonus, hyperreflexia, bilateral Babinski sign

Serotonin Syndrome

- Watch for patient on anti-depressants with fever, confusion, and rigid muscles
- Don't confuse with NMS
  - Both: muscle rigidity, fever, Δ MS, and autonomic instability
  - NMS: "Lead pipe" rigidity, ↑CK
  - SS: Clonus
- Treatment: cyproheptadine (5 –HT antagonist)

*fixed &
rigid
muscle
damages*

Acetylcholine

- Synthesized in basal nucleus of Meynert (subcortex)
- Increased levels in REM sleep
- Decreased levels in Alzheimer's
- Decreased levels in Huntington's disease

Glutamate –

- Major excitatory neurotransmitter
- N-methyl-D-aspartate (NMDA) receptor is target
- Huntington's: neuronal death from glutamate toxicity
  - Glutamate binds NMDA receptor
  - Excessive influx calcium
  - Cell death

Phencyclidine (PCP)
Angel Dust

- Antagonist to NMDA receptor
- Violent behavior
- Hallucinations
- Ataxia, nystagmus
- Hypertension, tachycardia, diaphoresis
- Can cause seizures, coma, or death

Dermatomes and Reflexes

Jason Ryan, MD, MPH

Dermatomes

C1 Nerve Root
C1 Vertebrae

C7
C7 Vertebrae
C8
T1 Vertebrae
T1
T2 Vertebrae

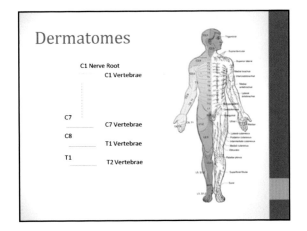

Key Spinal Nerves

- Phrenic nerve C3-C5
  - Innervates diaphragm
  - Diaphragm irritation → "referred" shoulder pain
  - Classic example is gallbladder disease
  - Also lower lung masses
  - Irritation can cause dyspnea and hiccups
  - Cut nerve → diaphragm elevation, dyspnea
- T10 = umbilicus
  - Referred pain for appendicitis

Herpes Zoster
Shingles

- Reactivation of latent varicella-zoster virus
  - Primary VZV = chicken pox
  - Fever, pharyngitis, vesicular rash
  - Shingles = reactivated VZV
- Lies dormant in dorsal root ganglia
- Rash along dermatome
- Does not cross midline
- Common in elderly or immunocompromised

Herpes Zoster

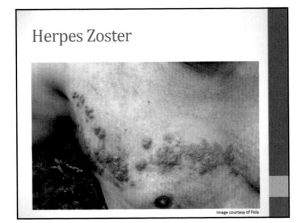

Image courtesy of Fisle

Reflexes

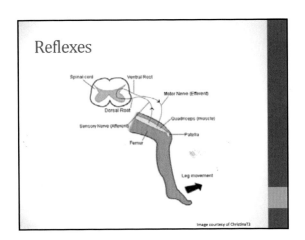

Image courtesy of ChristinaT3

Clinically Tested Reflexes

- Biceps – C5
- Triceps – C7
- Patella – L4
- Achilles (ankle jerk) – S1

Reflexes

- 0 = No reflex
- 1+ = diminished (LMN lesion)
- 2+ = Normal
- 3+ = Brisk (UMN lesion)
- 4+ = Very brisk
- 5+ = Sustained clonus

Nerve Root Syndromes

- L5 (L4/L5 disc)
  - Most common
  - Back pain down lat leg
  - Foot strength reduced
  - Reflexes normal
- S1 (L5/S1 disc)
  - 2nd most common
  - Pain down back of leg
  - Weakness plantar flexion
  - Ankle reflex lost

Babinski Sign
Plantar Reflex

- Rub bottom foot
- Normal: downward
  - Plantarflexion
- Abnormal: upward
  - Dorsiflexion
  - UMN damage
  - UMN suppress reflex
- Upward = normal infants
  - <12mo
  - Incomplete myelination

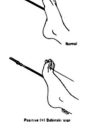

Normal

Positive (+) Babinski sign
(dorsiflexion of big toe)

Primitive Reflexes

- All present at birth in normal babies
- Disappear in first year of life or less
- Babies lacking these may have CNS pathology
- Reflexes that persist can indicate pathology
- Inhibited by mature frontal lobe
- Can reappear with frontal lobe pathology
- Six key reflexes:
  - Moro, Rooting, Sucking, Palmar, Plantar, Galant

Moro Reflex
Startle Reflex

- Lie baby on back
- Lift slightly off back
- Let go
- Three phase reflex
  - Spreading of arms
  - Unspreading of arms
  - Crying

Other Primitive Reflexes

- Rooting
  - Stroke cheek, baby turns toward side of stroke
- Sucking
  - Baby will suck anything touching roof of mouth
- Palmar
  - Stroke baby's palm, fingers will grasp
- Plantar
  - Babinski reflex → normal up to 1 year
- Galant
  - Stroke skin along babies back, baby swings legs to that side

Cerebral Cortex

Jason Ryan, MD, MPH

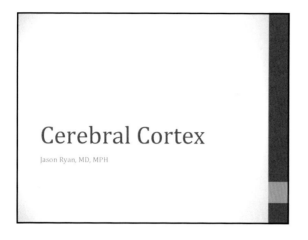

Cerebral Cortex

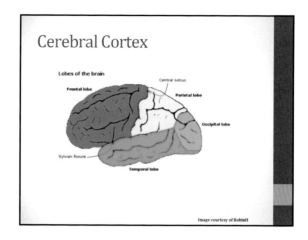

Image courtesy of RobinH

Brodmann areas

- 47 areas of human brain

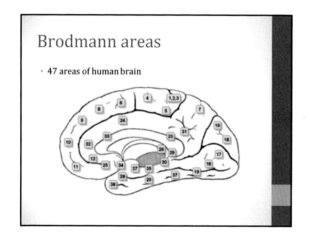

Frontal Lobe

- Largest lobe
- Motor function, planning movements
- Thinking, feeling, imagining, making decisions
- Key Areas
  - Motor cortex
  - Frontal Eye Fields
  - Broca's speech area
  - Prefrontal Cortex

Motor Cortex

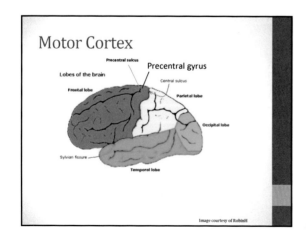

Image courtesy of RobinH

Homunculus

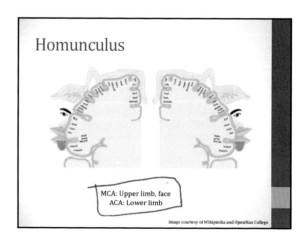

MCA: Upper limb, face
ACA: Lower limb

Image courtesy of Wikipiedia and OpenStax College

18

Frontal Eye Fields

- Found in frontal lobe
- Brodmann's Area 8
- Performs conjugate movement eyes to opposite side
- Saccadic movements: back-forth (reading)
- Complex function → helps track objects
- Destructive lesion:
  - Both eyes deviate to side of lesion

R   L

Right FEF Lesion

Broca's Speech Area

- Located in frontal lobe – LEFT hemisphere
- Speech production (not comprehension)
- Moves muscles for speech
- Makes speech clear, fluent
- Destruction → "expressive" aphasia
  - Know what you want to say but cannot express speech
  - Short sentences, stutters, stops
- Watch for "broken" speech: stuttering, stop/start

located near motor cortex

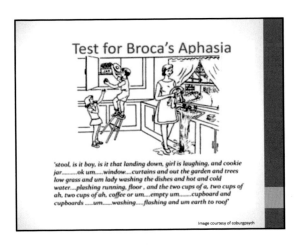

Test for Broca's Aphasia

'stool, is it boy, is it that landing down, girl is laughing, and cookie jar...........ok um......window....curtains and out the garden and trees low grass and um lady washing the dishes and hot and cold water....plashing running, floor , and the two cups of a, two cups of ah, two cups of ah, coffee or um....empty um.......cupboard and cupboards .....um......washing....flashing and um earth to roof'

Image courtesy of coburgpsych

Wernicke's Aphasia

- Located in temporal lobe – LEFT hemisphere
- Speech comprehension (not production)
- Destruction → "fluent" aphasia
  - Fluent, but meaningless speech
- Watch for LACK of stutters, starts/stops

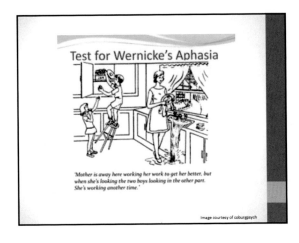

Test for Wernicke's Aphasia

'Mother is away here working her work to get her better, but when she's looking the two boys looking in the other part. She's working another time.'

Image courtesy of coburgpsych

Global Aphasia

- Both Broca's and Wernicke's (left side)
- Patient's often mute
- Cannot follow commands
- Can occur immediately following stroke
- Usually occurs with extensive CNS damage
  - Right Hemiparesis
  - Right visual loss

Prefrontal Cortex

- Anterior 2/3 of frontal lobe
- Lesions:
  - Disinhibition
  - Deficits in concentration
  - Disorientation
  - Poor judgment
  - Reemergence of primitive reflexes

Phineas Gage

- Railroad worker 1848
- Railroad iron thru skull
- Survived
- Personality change

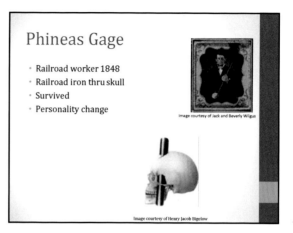

Image courtesy of Jack and Beverly Wilgus

Image courtesy of Henry Jacob Bigelow

Parietal Lobes

- Contain sensory cortex
- Damage to right parietal lobe: spatial neglect
  - Contralateral (left) agnosia
  - Can't perceive objects in part of space
  - Despite normal vision, somatic sensation
  - Failure to report or respond to stimuli affected side
- Right-sided spatial neglect rare
  - Redundant processing of right by left/right brain

Parietal Lobes

- Baum's Loop
- Part of visual pathway
- Damage: Quadrantic Anopia

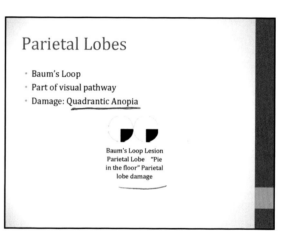

Baum's Loop Lesion
Parietal Lobe   "Pie
in the floor" Parietal
lobe damage

Temporal Lobe

- Primary auditory cortex
  - Lesions → "cortical" deafness
- Wernicke's speech area
  - Lesions → Wernicke's aphasia
- Olfactory bulb
- Meyer's Loop
- Hippocampus
- Amygdala

Olfactory Bulb

- Destruction → ipsilateral anosmia
- Psychomotor epilepsy
  - Sights, sounds, smells that are not there
  - Can result from irritation olfactory bulb
  - Part of temporal lobe epilepsy
- Rare, olfactory groove meningiomas
  - About 10% of all meningiomas
  - Cause anosmia

epilepsy

Meyer's Loop
Quadrantic Anopia

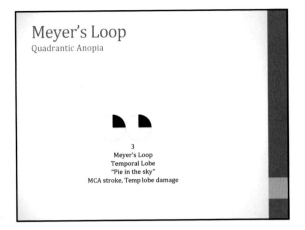

3
Meyer's Loop
Temporal Lobe
"Pie in the sky"
MCA stroke, Temp lobe damage

Amygdala

- Temporal lobe nuclei
- Important for decision making, higher functions
- Part of limbic system

Kluver-Bucy Syndrome

- Damage to bilateral amygdala (temporal lobes)
- Hyperphagia - Weight gain
- Hyperorality - tendency to examine all with mouth
- Inappropriate Sexual Behavior
  - Atypical sexual behavior, mounting inanimate objects
- Visual Agnosia
  - Inability to recognize visually presented objects
- Rare complication of HSV1 encephalitis

Occipital Lobe

- Vision
- Lesions cause cortical blindness
- Blood supply → PCA

Homonymous Hemianopsia

Left PCA Stroke
Right visual loss

Right PCA Stroke
Left visual loss

Macular Sparing

- Macula: central, high-resolution vision (reading)
- Dual blood supply: MCA and PCA
- PCA strokes often spare the macula

Spinal Cord

Jason Ryan, MD, MPH

Spine

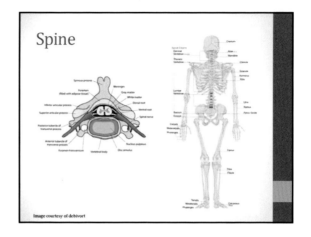

- Cervical (8)
- Thoracic (12)
- Lumbar (5)
- Sacral (5)
- Cord ends L1/L2
  - Conus medullaris
- Cauda Equina

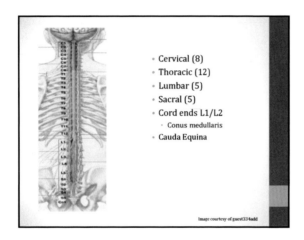

Spinal Cord Cross Section

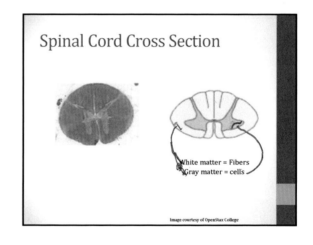

White matter = Fibers
Gray matter = cells

Spinal Cord Levels

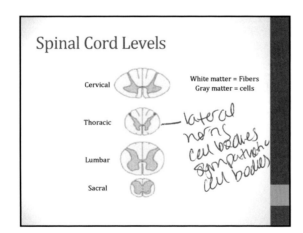

Cervical

White matter = Fibers
Gray matter = cells

Thoracic

lateral horns cell bodies sympathetic cell bodies

Lumbar

Sacral

Terminology

- Dorsal
  - Posterior
  - Towards Back
- Ventral
  - Anterior
  - Towards Front

- Rostral
  - Towards top of head
- Caudal
  - Towards tail
  - Away from head

Spinal Cord

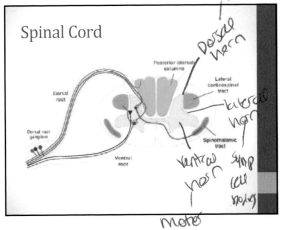

Handwritten annotations:
sensory spinothalamic tract
Dorsal horn
Lateral horn
Ventral horn — symp cell body
Motor

Spinal Cord Tracts

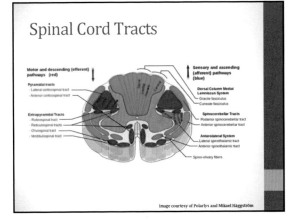

Image courtesy of Polarlys and Mikael Häggström

Spinal Cord

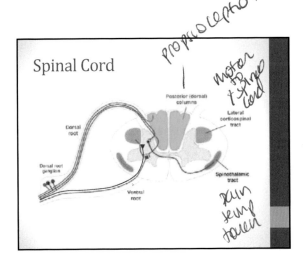

Handwritten annotations:
proprioception
motor to spinal cord
pain temp touch

Spinothalamic Tract
Pain/temperature/crude touch

1st Neuron: Spinal root to cord
2nd Neuron: Dorsal Horn
3rd Neuron: VPL Thalamus to Cortex

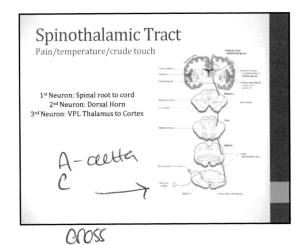

Handwritten annotations:
A - delta
C
cross

Spinothalamic Tract
Pain/temperature/crude touch

1st Neuron: Spinal root to cord
2nd Neuron: Dorsal Horn to Thalamus
3rd Neuron: VPL Thalamus to Cortex

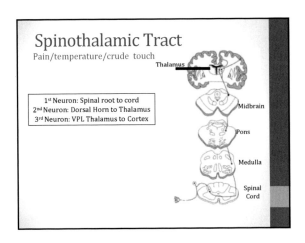

Thalamus
Midbrain
Pons
Medulla
Spinal Cord

Posterior Column
Dorsal Column-Medial Lemniscus

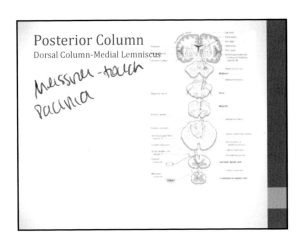

Handwritten annotations:
Meissner - touch
Pacinia

Posterior Column
Dorsal Column-Medial Lemniscus

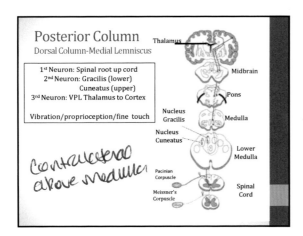

1st Neuron: Spinal root up cord
2nd Neuron: Gracilis (lower)
Cuneatus (upper)
3rd Neuron: VPL Thalamus to Cortex
Vibration/proprioception/fine touch

(handwritten) Contralateral above medulla

Sensory Info to Brain

- Spinothalamic
  - Pain/temperature/crude touch
  - Synapse cord level
  - Cross cord level
- Posterior column
  - Vibration/proprioception/fine touch
  - Ascend in cord
  - Synapse nucleus gracilis/cuneatus
  - Cross medulla
- Key point: Both cross but in different places

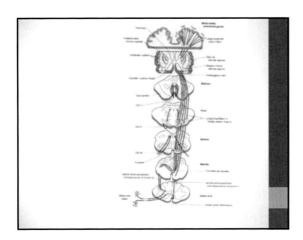

Corticospinal Tract

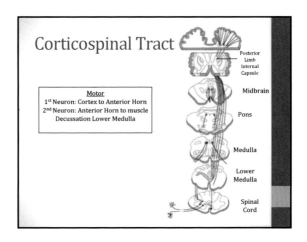

Motor
1st Neuron: Cortex to Anterior Horn
2nd Neuron: Anterior Horn to muscle
Decussation Lower Medulla

Key Points

1. Anterior Horn – Motor nerves
2. Posterior Horn – Sensory Nerves (pain/temp)
3. Lateral Horn – Autonomic Nerves *(handwritten)* only thoracic
4. Spinothalamic Tract – Pain/Temp
5. Medial lemniscus – Vibration/Proprioception *(handwritten)* posterior column
6. Corticospinal Tract - Motor

Testing Sensation

- Romberg
  - Positive suggests posterior column problem
- Vibration
  - Tuning fork
- Proprioception
  - Close eyes; "Is toe up or down?"

Testing Sensation

- Pain
  - Pin prick
- Temp
  - Hot/cold water (rarely done)

Peripheral Neuropathy

- Diabetes complication
  - Pin prick weak at feet, better further up leg
  - Changes with going up the leg
  - Not spinal cord problem

Spinal Cord Syndromes

Jason Ryan, MD, MPH

Spinal Cord Syndromes

1. Poliomyelitis and Werdnig-Hoffman disease
2. Multiple sclerosis
3. Amyotrophic lateral sclerosis (ALS)
4. Anterior spinal artery occlusion
5. Tabes dorsalis
6. Syringomyelia
7. Subacute combined degeneration (SCD)

Polio

- Single stranded RNA virus
- Prevented by vaccination
- Destruction of anterior horn
- LMN lesions
- Flaccid paralysis

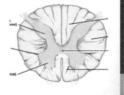

Polio

- Classic presentation
  - Unvaccinated child
  - Febrile illness
  - Neuro symptoms 4-5 days later
  - Weakness (legs>arms)
  - Flaccid muscle tone

Werdnig-Hoffman Disease

- Spinal muscle atrophy disease
- Hypotonia/weakness in newborn
- Classic finding: tongue fasciculations
- "Floppy baby"
- Similar lesions to polio *anterior motor horn*
- Death in few months

Multiple Sclerosis

- Mostly cervical white matter
- Random, asymmetric lesions
- Relapsing, remitting pattern

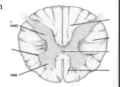

young women

Amyotrophic lateral sclerosis

- Combined UMN/LMN disease
- No sensory symptoms!!
- Upper symptoms
  - Spasticity, exaggerated reflexes
- Lower symptoms
  - Wasting, fasciculations

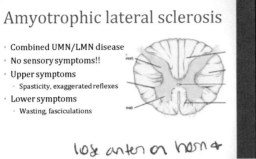

lose anterior horn + corticalspinal tract

Amyotrophic lateral sclerosis

- Cranial nerves can be involved
  - Dysphagia
- Most common 40-60 years old
- Usually fatal 3-5 years
- Common cause of death: aspiration pneumonia
- Riluzole for treatment (↓glutamate release neurons)

Amyotrophic lateral sclerosis

- Familial cases:
  - Zinc copper superoxide dismutase deficiency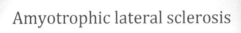
  - Increased free radical damage

Lou Gehrig

- Baseball player
- NY Yankees 1930s
- The Iron Horse

Amyotrophic lateral sclerosis

- Classic Presentation
  - 50-year old patient
  - Slowly progressive course
  - Arm weakness
  - Dysphagia to solids/liquids
  - Some flaccid muscles
  - Some spastic muscles
  - No sensory symptoms

ASA Occlusion

- Loss of all but posterior columns
- Only vibration, proprioception intact
- Acute onset (stroke)
- Flaccid bilateral paralysis (loss of LMN) below lesion

posterior column spared

lose Bilat motor/sens

intact vibration/proprioception

Tabes dorsalis

- Tertiary syphilis
- Demyelination of posterior columns
- Loss of dorsal roots

↓ proprioception
↓ reflexes

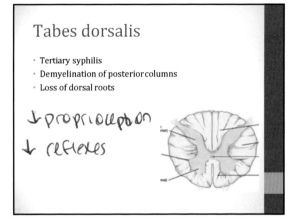

Tabes dorsalis

- Classic Signs/Symptoms
  - Patient with other STDs
  - Difficulty walking
  - 5/5 strength legs and arms
  - Positive Romberg (no proprio)
  - Wide-based gate
  - Fleeting, recurrent shooting pains
  - Loss of ankle/knee reflexes
  - Argyll Robertson pupils

↳ small, no light but accommodates

Syringomyelia

- Fluid-filled space in spinal canal
- Damages ST nerve fibers crossing center
- Bilateral loss pain/temp
- Usually C8-T1 (arms/hands)

arms &
hands

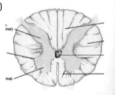

Syringomyelia

- Can expand to affect anterior horn
  - Muscle weakness
- Can expand to affect lateral horn
  - Loss of sympathetic to face
  - Horner's syndrome
- Can cause kyphoscoliosis (spine curve)

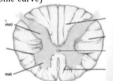

Syringomyelia

- From trauma or congenital
- Can occur years after spinal cord injury
- Seen in Chiari malformations

Syringomyelia

- Symptoms only at level of the syrinx
- Usually C8-T1
  - Watch for pin prick/temp loss on only hands/back
  - Legs will be normal
- Position, vibration normal all levels
- Temp loss may present as burns not felt
- Pain loss may present as cuts not felt
- If large, motor symptoms may develop
- If large, Horner's syndrome may develop

Syringomyelia

- Classic presentation
  - Cuts/burns on hands that were not felt
  - Loss of pinprick and temp in back, shoulders, arms
- May also include:
  - Motor weakness arms
  - Horner's syndrome

SCD

- B12 Deficiency
- Demyelination posterior columns (vibr/proprio)
- Loss of lateral motor tracts
- Slowly progressive
- Weakness
- Ataxia
- May not have macrocytosis

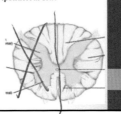

SCD

- Classic presentation
  - Problems walking
  - Positive Romberg
  - Spastic paresis in legs
  - Lower extremity hyperreflexia
  - Positive Babinski

Brown-Sequard Syndrome

- Loss of half of spinal cord
- Trauma or tumor
- Lose pain/temp contralateral side
- Lose motor, position, vibration ipsilateral side

Below Level of Injury

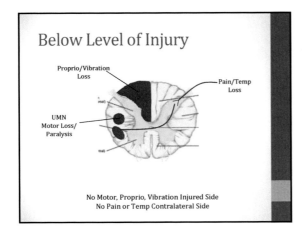

No Motor, Proprio, Vibration Injured Side
No Pain or Temp Contralateral Side

Level of Injury

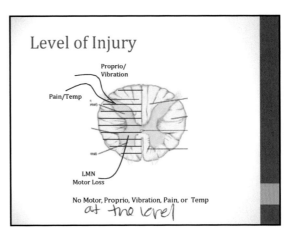

No Motor, Proprio, Vibration, Pain, or Temp

at the level

UMN below

Brown-Sequard Syndrome

- Weak side = side with lesion
- UMN signs below
- 1: Level of lesion
  - LMN signs
  - Loss of all sensation
  - If above T1 → Horner's
  - Constricted pupil, eyelid droop
- 2: Loss of motor, posterior columns
- 3: Loss of pain/temp

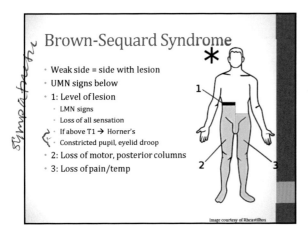

Image courtesy of Rhcastilhos

Brown-Sequard Syndrome

- Classic Presentation
  - Prior trauma (knife, gunshot)
  - Level of injury: No sensation
  - Side with injury
    - Spastic paresis; Babinski sign
    - Loss of vibration/proprioception
  - Other side
    - Loss of pain/temp

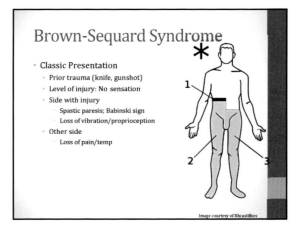

Image courtesy of Rhcastilhos

Cauda Equina Syndrome

- Spinal cord ends about L2 (conus medullaris)
- Spinal nerves continue inferiorly (cauda equina)
- Cauda equina nerve roots:
  - Motor to lower extremity
  - Sensory to lower extremity
  - Pelvic floor/sphincter innervation
- Cauda equina syndrome:
  - Compression cauda equina
  - Massive disk rupture
  - Trauma, tumor

Cauda Equina Syndrome

- Classic Presentation
  - Severe low back pain
  - "Saddle anesthesia"
  - Loss of anocutaneous reflex
  - Bowel and bladder dysfunction
  - Normal Babinski

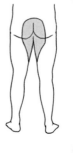

Image courtesy of Lesion

Conus Medullaris Syndrome

- Perianal anesthesia, bilateral
- Impotence

Brainstem

Jason Ryan, MD, MPH

Terminology

- Dorsal
  - Posterior
  - Towards Back
- Ventral
  - Anterior
  - Towards Front
- Rostral
  - Towards top of head
- Caudal
  - Towards tail
  - Away from head

The Brainstem

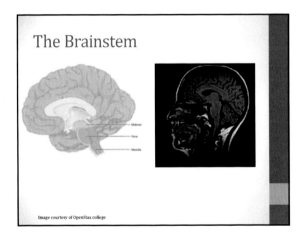

Image courtesy of OpenStax college

The Brainstem

- Sensory and motor fibers
- Nuclei of cranial nerves
- Important to know what lies in each section
  - Midbrain
  - Pons
  - Medulla
- Focus on
  - Which cranial nerves each level?
  - Where are the tracts traveling btw brain/cord?
  - Medial versus lateral?

Brainstem Sections

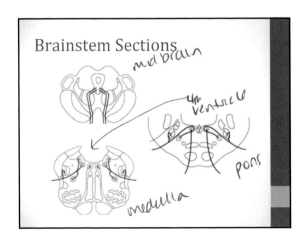

Midbrain
Mesencephalon

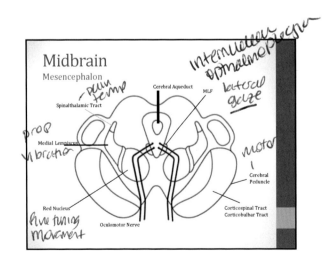

31

Benedikt Syndrome

- CN 3, medial leminiscus, red nucleus
- Oculomotor palsy — *Down + out*
- Contralateral loss proprioception/vibration
- Involuntary movements
  - Tremor
  - Ataxia

Weber's Syndrome

- CN3, corticospinal tract, corticobulbar tract
- Occulomotor nerve palsy
- Contralateral hemiparesis
- Pseudobulbar palsy
  - UMN cranial nerve motor weakness
  - Exaggerated gag reflex
  - Tongue spastic (no wasting)
  - Spastic dysarthria

Parinaud's Syndrome

- Posterior midbrain
- Superior colliculus and pretectal area
  - Can't look up (vertical gaze palsy)
- Pseudo Argyll Robertson pupil
- Often from pinealoma/germinoma of pineal region
- Watch for cerebral aqueduct obstruction
  - Non-communicating hydrocephalus
  - Compression from a pineal tumor

Pons

Facial sensation

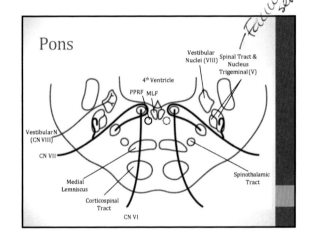

Medial Pontine Syndromes

- Corticospinal tract, CN 6, CN 7
- Contralateral hemiparesis
- CN 6 palsy
- Facial weakness/droop affected side
- Lateral gaze structures: MLF, CN VI nucleus
- Gaze palsies
  - Can't look to affected side
  - Damage to either PPRF or nucleus CN VI

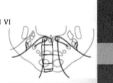

Lateral Pontine Syndromes

- Vestibular nuclei: nystagmus, vertigo, N/V
- Spinothalamic tract: Contralateral pain/temp
- Spinal V nucleus: ipsilateral face pain/temp
- Sympathetic tract: Horner's syndrome
- Facial nucleus:
  - Ipsilateral facial droop
  - Loss corneal reflex
- Cochlear nuclei
  - Deafness
- AICA stroke

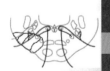

Medulla

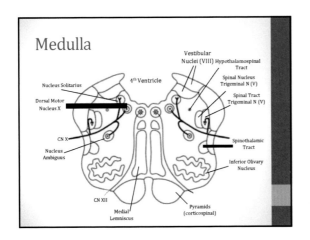

Nucleus Solitarius
Dorsal Motor Nucleus X
CN X
Nucleus Ambiguus
4ᵗʰ Ventricle
Vestibular Nuclei (VIII) Hypothalamospinal Tract
Spinal Nucleus Trigeminal N (V)
Spinal Tract Trigeminal N (V)
Spinothalamic Tract
Inferior Olivary Nucleus
CN XII
Medial Lemniscus
Pyramids (corticospinal)

Medial Medullary Syndrome

- Corticospinal, medial lemniscus, CN 12
- Contralateral Hemiparesis
- Contralateral loss of proprioception/vibration
- Flaccid paralysis tongue
  - Deviation to side of lesion
- Anterior spinal artery stroke

Lateral Medullary Syndrome
Wallenberg's Syndrome

- Vestibular nuclei: Nystagmus, vertigo, N/V
- Sympathetic tract: Horner's syndrome
- Spinothalamic tract: Contralateral pain/temp
- Spinal V nucleus: ipsilateral face pain/temp
- Nucleus ambiguus (IX, X)
  - Hoarseness, dysphagia
- PICA Stroke

How to Find Lesions

- Option 1: Know the syndromes
- Option 2: Use the Rule of 4s

Rule of 4s

- 4 CNs in:
  - Medulla
  - Pons
  - Above Pons
- 4 CNs divide into 12
  - III, IV, VI, XII
  - Motor nuclei are midline
- 4 CNs do not divide/12
  - V, VII, IX, XI
  - All are lateral

- 4 midline columns
  - Motor nucleus
  - Motor pathway
  - MLF
  - Medial Lemniscus
- 4 lateral (side) columns
  - Sympathetic
  - Spinothalamic
  - Sensory
  - Spinocerebellar

Dr. Peter Gates. The rule of 4 of the brainstem: a simplified method for understanding brainstem anatomy and brainstem vascular syndromes for the non-neurologist. Internal Medicine Journal Volume 35, Issue 4, pages 263–266, April 2005

Localizing Lesions

- Medial vs. Lateral
  - Which tracts affected?
- Medulla vs. Pons vs. Midbrain
  - Which cranial nerves affected?

Midbrain
Pons
Medulla
CNs
Tracts
Media ---------- Lateral

4 Above Pons CNs

	Deficit
Olfactory CN1	Not in midbrain
Optic CN2	Not in midbrain
Oculomotor CN3	Eye turned out and down
Trochlear CN4	Eye unable to look down when looking towards nose

4 Pons CNs

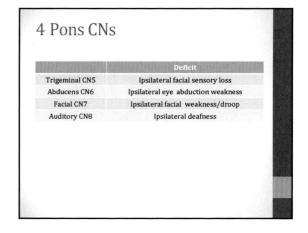

	Deficit
Trigeminal CN5	Ipsilateral facial sensory loss
Abducens CN6	Ipsilateral eye abduction weakness
Facial CN7	Ipsilateral facial weakness/droop
Auditory CN8	Ipsilateral deafness

4 Medulla CNs

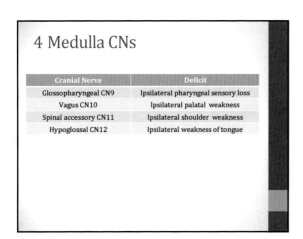

Cranial Nerve	Deficit
Glossopharyngeal CN9	Ipsilateral pharyngeal sensory loss
Vagus CN10	Ipsilateral palatal weakness
Spinal accessory CN11	Ipsilateral shoulder weakness
Hypoglossal CN12	Ipsilateral weakness of tongue

Midline Structures (M)

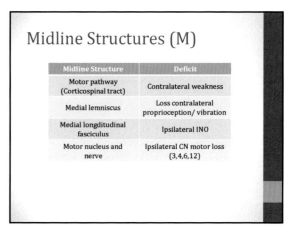

Midline Structure	Deficit
Motor pathway (Corticospinal tract)	Contralateral weakness
Medial lemniscus	Loss contralateral proprioception/ vibration
Medial longditudinal fasciculus	Ipsilateral INO
Motor nucleus and nerve	Ipsilateral CN motor loss (3,4,6,12)

Side/Lateral Structures (S)

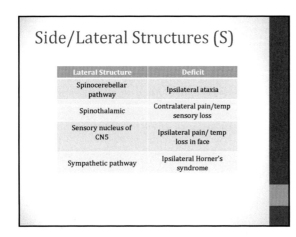

Lateral Structure	Deficit
Spinocerebellar pathway	Ipsilateral ataxia
Spinothalamic	Contralateral pain/temp sensory loss
Sensory nucleus of CN5	Ipsilateral pain/ temp loss in face
Sympathetic pathway	Ipsilateral Horner's syndrome

Rule of 4s Caveats

- Trigeminal Nerve (V)
  - Lesion: loss of ipsilateral pain/temp face
  - Rule of 4 Pons Nuclei and side (lateral tract)
  - Don't use to localize to Pons
  - Use for lateral tract localization
- Vestibulocochlear (VIII)
  - Don't use vestibular sings to localize to pons
  - Vestibular signs can be medulla/pons
  - Lesion: hearing loss

Case 1

- A 75-year-old man presents for evaluation of weakness. He reports that two hours ago he suddenly was unable to move his left arm or leg. He denies any difficulty with speech. On examination, he is able to move all facial muscles normally. There is no ophthalmoplegia. On tongue protrusion, the tongue is deviated to the right. He in unable to detect lower or upper extremity vibration on the left.

Case 1

- Complete motor weakness
  - Not MCA or ACA stroke
- Tongue involved: brainstem lesion
- Motor pathway involved – left side weak
  - Right medial lesion
- Medial lemniscus involved left (vibration/prop)
  - Right medial lesion
- CN XII involved – tongue deviation
  - Medulla
- Answer: Right medial medullary syndrome
- Anterior spinal artery

Brainstem Blood Supply

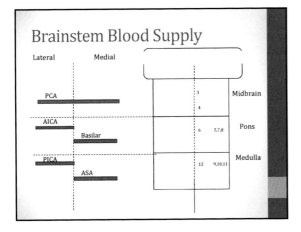

Lateral   Medial

PCA

AICA

Basilar

PICA

ASA

3
4   Midbrain

6   5,7,8   Pons

12   9,10,11   Medulla

Case 2

- Right sided weakness
- Left eye down/out, dilated

Case 2

- Right sided weakness
  - Motor pathway
  - Medial lesion
  - Complete motor loss: not MCA, ACA
- Left eye down/out, dilated
  - CNIII
- Left medial midbrain lesion
- Weber's syndrome
- Stroke of branches of PCA

Case 3

- Unable to do left hand finger to nose test
- Loss of pain and temperature to left face
- Left eyelid droop, small pupil
- Loss of pain/temp right arm and leg
- Hoarse voice
- Loss of gag reflex left throat
- Palate raised on right side

Case 3

- Unable to do left hand finger to nose test — Left ataxia
- Loss of pain and temperature to left face — Left CN V
- Left eyelid droop, small pupil — Left Horner's
- Loss of pain/temp right arm and leg — Left ST Tract
- Hoarse voice — CN X
- Loss of gag reflex left throat — CN IX
- Palate raised on right side — CN X

Case 3

- Left ataxia = spinocerebellar
- Left face pain/temp = sensory (CN V) face
- Left Horner's = sympathetic
- Right pain/temp = left spinothalamic
- Speaking, gag, palate = CN IX, X
- Left lateral medulla
- Wallenberg's syndrome
- Left PICA stroke

Case 4

- Right deafness/tinnitus
- Loss right finger to nose
- Right facial numbness
- No corneal reflex
- Right facial spasms

Case 4

- Right deafness/tinnitus — Right VIII Right
- Loss right finger to nose — spinocerebellar Right
- Right facial numbness — sensory
- No corneal reflex — Right CN V
- Right facial spasms — Right CN VII

Right Lateral Pons Cerebellopontine
angle syndrome Often caused by tumors
(schwannomas)

Rule of 4s

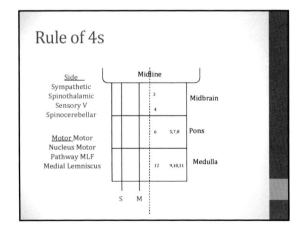

Brainstem Blood Supply

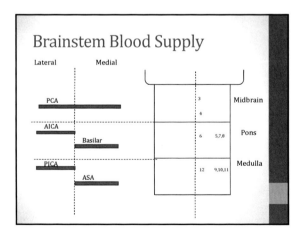

36

Cranial Nerves

Jason Ryan, MD, MPH

Cranial Nerves

- 12 nerves with roots in brainstem and CNS
- Sensory, Motor, Visceral
- Things to know:
  - Sensory vs. Motor vs. Both
  - Special features
  - Lesions

Olfactory (I)x

- Smell (sensory)
- Pathway: cribriform plate of ethmoid bone
- Synapse in olfactory bulb → piriform cortex
- Lesions: anosmia
- Only sensory nerve no thalamus input
- Damage by trauma
  - Skull fracture
- Rarely infections or tumors

Optic (II)

Right Optic Nerve Compression

- Sight (sensory)
- Pathway: optic canal of the sphenoid bone
- Not really a peripheral nerve
- Arises from diencephalon
  - Embryonic structure
  - In adults: upper end of brain stem
  - Thalamus, hypothalamus
- Only CN I & II found outside brainstem

Oculomotor (III)

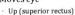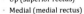

- Moves eye
  - Up (superior rectus)
  - Medial (medial rectus)
  - Inferior (inferior rectus)
  - Superior rotation (inferior oblique)
- Elevates eyelid (levator palpebrae)
- Pupillary constriction (sphincter pupillae)
- Palsy: eye down, out, pupil dilated, ptosis

Trochlear(IV)

- Eye movement (motor)
- Smallest cranial nerve
- Superior oblique
  - Turns eye down/in
  - Reading/stairs
- Palsy symptoms
  - Diplopia
  - Eye tilted outward
  - Unable to look down/in (stairs, reading)
  - Head tilting away from affected side (to compensate)

Trigeminal (V)

- Sensory and Motor
- Key function: Sensor (touch-pain-temp) to face
- Largest cranial nerve
- 3 divisions: ophthalmic, maxillary, mandibular
  - V1, V2, V3
- 3 important functions:
  - Part of corneal reflex (sensory, V1)
  - Muscles of mastication (chewing)

Trigeminal (V)

- Palsy
  - Numb face
  - Weak jaw → deviates to affected side
    - Unopposed action of normal side
- Trigeminal neuralgia
  - Recurrent, sudden sharp pains in half of face
  - Tic douloureux (painful tic)
  - So intense you wince ("tic")
  - Treatment: Carbamazepine

Corneal Reflex

- Touch eye with Q-tip
- Sensed by V1 of CN V
- Transmit to VII (bilaterally)
- CNVII → blink
- Key points:
  - Need CN V for sense
  - Need CN VII for blinking

Abducens (VI)

- Eye movement (motor)
- Lateral rectus
- Palsy
  - Diplopia
  - Can't laterally move (look out) affected eye

Facial (VII)

- Motor, sensory
- Muscles of facial expression
- Taste, salivation, lacrimation
- Some ear muscles
- Special feature
  - Dual UMN innervation

Lower Facial Droop

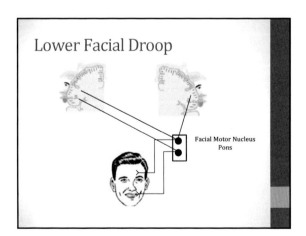

Facial Motor Nucleus
Pons

Lower Facial Droop

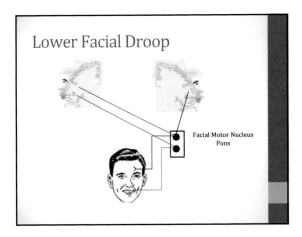

Facial Motor Nucleus
Pons

Lower Facial Droop

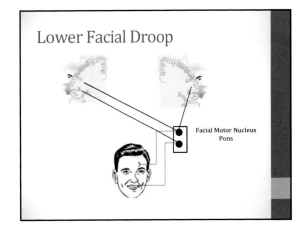

Facial Motor Nucleus
Pons

Lower Facial Droop

- UMN damage (MCA Stroke)
  - Upper face intact (dual supply)
  - Lower face affected
- LMN damage
  - Whole half of face affected

Facial (VII)

- Palsy
  - Loss of corneal reflex (motor part)
  - Loss of taste anterior 2/3 tongue
  - Hyperacusis (stapedius paralysis)
    - Pt cannot tolerate sounds

Bell's Palsy

- Idiopathic mononeuropathy of CN VII
- Facial paralysis
- Usually resolves in weeks to months
- Thought to be due to HSV-1 induced nerve damage
- Other causes of CN VII neuropathy (technically not BP)
  - Lyme
  - Tumor
  - Stroke

Vestibulocochlear (VIII)

- Sensory
- Equilibrium, balance, hearing
- Vestibular portion
  - Compensatory eye movements
  - Lesions: vertigo, nystagmus, disequilibrium
- Cochlear portion
  - Hearing
  - Lesions: tinnitus, hearing loss

Testing CN VIII

- Awake patient
  - Ask them to focus eyes on object while you rotate head
  - If eyes stay fixed→ both CN VIII are working
  - "Doll's eyes" → CN VIII lesion
  - When head rotate toward lesion side, eye moves with head then quickly adjusts when the head stops moving (saccade)

Testing CN VIII

- Unconscious patient
- Inject cold water into ear
  - Cold water disrupts CN VIII function
  - Eyes slowly move toward cold water
  - Rapid correct opposite side
  - Normal response is slow toward cold then fast away
  - If CN VIII not working, no slow toward
  - If cortex not working, slow toward, no fast away

Testing CN VIII

- Unconscious patient
- Inject warm water into ear
  - Warm water stimulates CN VIII function
  - Creates "relative" opposite side CN VIII dysfunction
  - Eyes slowly move away warm water
  - Rapid correct back towards warm water
  - Normal response is slow away then fast toward
  - If CN VIII not working, no slow away
  - If cortex not working, slow away, no fast toward

Testing CN VIII

- COWS: Cold Opposite, Warm Same
  - Named for side of fast correction
- Easy way:
  - If warm or cold water in ear yields no eye response, lesion is on that side

Glossopharyngeal (IX)

- Motor, Sensory
- Taste/sensation posterior 1/3 tongue
- Swallowing
- Salivation (parotid gland)
- Carotid body and sinus
  - Chemo- and baroreceptors
- Stylopharyngeus (elevates pharynx)

Glossopharyngeal (IX)

- Palsy
  - Loss of gag reflex
  - Loss of taste posterior 1/3 tongue
  - Loss sensation upper pharynx/tonsils
- Hemodynamic effects
  - Tricks body into thinking low BP
  - ↑HR, Vasoconstriction, ↑BP

Vagus (X)

- Motor, sensory
- Taste epiglottis
- Swallowing (dysphagia = vagus)
- Palate elevation
- Midline uvula
- Talking
- Coughing
- Autonomic system
  - Aortic arch chemo/baroreceptors

Vagus (X)

- Palsy
  - Hoarseness, dysphagia, dysarthria
  - Loss of gag reflex
  - Loss of sensation pharynx and larynx
  - Weak side of palate collapses (lower)
  - Uvula deviates AWAY from affected side
- Hemodynamic effects
  - Unopposed sympathetic stim of heart
  - Result is ↑HR

Cranial Nerve Speech Test

- "Kuh kuh kuh"
  - CN X
  - Raise palate
- "Mi mi mi"
  - CN VII
  - Move lips
- "La La La"
  - CN XII
  - Move tongue

Recurrent Laryngeal Nerve

- Branch of vagus
- Ascends towards larynx between trachea/esophagus
  - "tracheoesophageal groove"
- Right RL: loops around R subclav
  Left RL: loops around aortic arch
- Compression → hoarseness
- Dilated left atrium (mitral stenosis)
- Aortic dissection

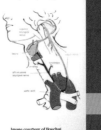

Image courtesy of Jkwchui

Vasovagal Syncope

- Most common cause of syncope (fainting)
- Trigger to vagus nerve
  - Increased parasympathetic outflow via vagus
- ↓HR ↓BP → fainting
- Many triggers
  - Hot weather
  - Prolonged standing
  - Pain
  - Sight of blood

Accessory (XI)

- Motor
- Turning head
- Shoulder shrugging
  - Sternocleidomastoid
  - Trapezius

Accessory (XI)

- Palsy
  - Difficulty turning head toward normal side (SCM)
  - Shoulder droop (affected side)

Hypoglossal (XII)

- Motor
- Tongue movement
- Palsy:
  - Protrusion of tongue TOWARD affected side
  - Opposite side pushes tongue away unopposed

Cranial Nerve Reflexes

- Corneal
  - V1 sense, VII blinking
- Lacrimation
  - V1 sense, VII for tearing
  - Cut V1 → No reflex tears, Yes emotional tears
- Gag
  - IX sense, X gag

Cranial Nerve Reflexes

- Jaw Jerk
  - Place finger patient's chin and tap finger
  - Jaw will jerk upwards
  - V3 sense, V3 jerk (Trigeminal nerve test)
- Pupillary
  - II senses light
  - III constricts pupil

Tongue

- Motor:
  - Hypoglossal (XII)
  - Lesion deviates tongue to affected side
  - One exception: palatoglossus (CN X)
- General Sensory (pain, pressure, temp, touch)
  - Anterior 2/3: Mandibular branch (CN V3)
  - Posterior 1/3: Glossopharyngeal (IX)
  - Tongue root: CN X
- Taste
  - Anterior 2/3: CN VII
  - Posterior 1/3: Glossopharyngeal (IX)
  - Tongue root, larynx, upper esophagus: CN X
- Terminal sulcus separates ant 2/3 from post 1/3

Cranial Nerve Skull Pathways

- Cribriform plate – CN I
- Middle cranial fossa – CN II-VI
  - CNII: Optic canal
  - III, IV, V1, VI: Superior orbital fossa
  - V2: Foramen rotundum
  - V3: Foramen Ovale
- Posterior cranial fossa – CN VII-XII
  - VII, VIII: Internal auditory meatus
  - IX, X, XI: Jugular foramen
  - Foramen magnum: XI (also brainstem)
  - XII: Hypoglossal canal

Image courtesy of Anatomist90

Auditory System

Jason Ryan, MD, MPH

How We Hear

- Sound waves cause tympanic membrane vibration
- Malleus, incus, stapes
  - Tiny bones
  - Amplify tympanic membrane motion
- Stapes pushes fluid-filled cochlea
- Tiny hair cells stimulated
  - Organ of Corti
  - Different frequencies of sound move different fibers
- Nerve (electrical) signal generated

The Inner Ear

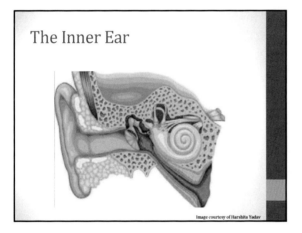

Image courtesy of Harshita Yadav

Auditory Pathway

- Cochlear nerve (CN VIII)
- Cerebellopontine angle
  - Lateral Pons
  - Watch for brainstem lesions with hearing loss
- Connects with many structures
  - Superior olivary nucleus
  - Trapezoid body
  - Lateral lemniscus
  - Inferior colliculus
  - Medial geniculate body
  - Transverse temporal gyri of Heschl

Types of Hearing Loss

- Conductive
  - Sound waves can't covert to nerve signals
  - Obstruction (wax)
  - Infection (otitis media)
  - Otosclerosis (bony overgrowth of stapes)
- Sensorineural
  - Cochlea disease
  - Cochlear nerve failure (acoustic neuroma)
  - CN damage

Presbycusis

- Age-related hearing loss
- Degeneration of Organ of Corti
- Results in sensorineural hearing loss
- Slow development over time

Weber Test

- Vibrating tuning fork
- Bridge of the forehead, nose, or teeth
- Should be equal in both ears

Weber Test

Normal	Conductive	Sensorineural
Signal equal both ears	Louder bad ear No background noise	Louder good ear No nerve to sense vibration

If sound goes to one side, tells you there is a hearing defect
Does not tell you which type

Rinne Test

- Tuning fork placed mastoid bone (behind the ear)
  - Tests bone conduction => vibration waves through bone
- Wait until patient no longer hears
- Move tuning fork to just outside ear
  - Tests air conduction only
- Ask if patient can still hear

Rinne Test

- Normal patient can still hear next to ear
  - AC > BC
- Conductive Loss
  - Patient CANNOT hear next to ear
  - AC<BC
- Sensorineural loss
  - Patient can still hear next to ear
  - Both AC and BC reduced
  - AC still > BC

Diagnosing Hearing Loss

Test	Conductive	Sensorineural
Weber	Louder bad ear	Louder good ear
Rinne	AC<BC bad ear	AC>BC bad ear

Normal
AC>BC
Weber Equal

Audiometry

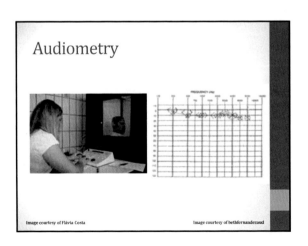

Image courtesy of Flávia Costa   Image courtesy of bethfernandezaud

Noise-induced Hearing Loss

- Sudden after loud noise
  - Tympanic membrane rupture
- Long term noise exposure
  - Damage to ciliated (hair) cells Organ of Corti
  - High-frequency hearing lost first

Vestibular System

Jason Ryan, MD, MPH

The Inner Ear

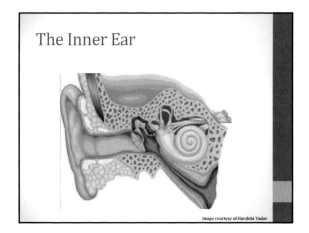

Image courtesy of Harshita Yadav

Vestibular System

- Vestibule: Central portion inner ear
- Found within temporal bone
- Contains system for balance, posture, equilibrium
- Also coordinates head and eye movements

Vestibular System

- Three semicircular canals (x, y, z planes of motion)
  - Respond to ROTATION of head
  - Filled with endolymph
  - Bulges at base (ampulla)
  - Ampulla have hair cells that bend with rotation
  - Hair cells release neurotransmitters → action potential
  - More/less signals based on motion

Vestibular System

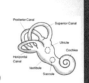

- Utricle and saccule (otolith organs)
  - Respond to LINEAR motion
  - Gravity, moving forward/backward
  - Contain otoliths (Greek word: ear stones)
  - Calcium carbonate crystals
  - Sit on top of hair cells
  - Drag hair cells in response to motion
  - This generates vestibular neural activity

Vestibular Nerve Signals

- Vestibulocochlear nerve
  - Two nerves in 1 sheath: Vestibular & Cochlear
- Vestibular nerve
  - Send signals to brainstem (vestibular nuclei)
  - Also sends signals to Cerebellum
- Vestibular nuclei
  - Beneath floor of 4th ventricle in pons/medulla
  - Receive input from vestibular nerve
  - Many outputs: Cerebellum, CNs III, IV, VI, Thalamus

Vestibular Dysfunction

- Vertigo: Room spinning when head still
  - Contrast with dizzy, lightheaded
- Nystagmus : Rhythmic oscillation of eyes
- Nausea/vomiting

Nystagmus

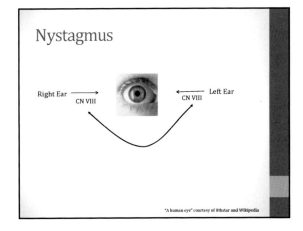

Right Ear —→ CN VIII   ←— CN VIII   Left Ear

"A human eye" courtesy of 8thstar and Wikipedia

Nystagmus

- Vestibulo-ocular reflex
- Focuses eyes when body moves
- Vestibular dysfunction → disrupts reflex
- Eyes move slowly one direction → fast correction
- "Jerk" nystagmus named for fast direction
  - Left
  - Right
  - Torsional/rotational
  - Upbeat
  - Downbeat
- Pendular nystagmus – Rare, congenital

Nystagmus

- Left, right, torsional/rotational
  - Seen with "peripheral" vestibular dysfunction
- Upbeat, downbeat
  - Seen with "central" vestibular dysfunction

Central vs. Peripheral
Nystagmus/Vertigo

- Peripheral = Benign (usually)
  - Inner ear problem
  - Benign positional vertigo (BPV)
  - Vestibular neuritis
  - Meniere's disease
- Central = BAD
  - Brainstem or cerebellar lesion
  - Vertebrobasilar stroke/TIA
  - Cerebellar infarction/hemorrhage
  - Tumor (posterior fossa)

Clinical Features

- Central Vertigo
  - Purely vertical nystagmus
  - Nystagmus changes direction with gaze
  - Positional testing: IMMEDIATE nystagmus
  - Skew deviation: Vertical misalignment of eyes
  - Diplopia, Dysmetria (ataxia)
  - Other CNS symptoms (weakness, sensory)

Clinical Features

- Peripheral Features
  - Mixed horizontal/torsional nystagmus
  - Positional testing: DELAYED nystagmus
  - Nystagmus may fatigues with time
  - No other symptoms
  - Normal proprioception, stable Romberg

Dix-Hallpike Maneuver

- Done to reproduce vertigo and cause nystagmus
- Seated patient
- Extend neck, turn head to side
- Rapidly lie patient down on table
- Let head hang over end of table

Dix-Hallpike Maneuver

- Typical result in BPV
  - No symptoms for 5-10 seconds
  - Vertigo develops
  - Torsional nystagmus develops
  - Symptoms resolve with sitting up
  - Fewer symptoms with repeated maneuvers

Benign Positional Vertigo

- Vertigo with head turning/position
- Due to calcium debris semicircular canals
  - Canalithiasis
- Diagnosis: Dix Hallpike Maneuver
- Deviations from typical result = consider imaging
- Epley Maneuver can reposition otoconia

Vestibular Neuronitis
Labyrinthitis

- Cause of vertigo
- Neuropathy of vestibular portion CN VIII
- Benign, self-limited
- Usually viral or post-inflammatory

Meniere's Disease

- Endolymph fluid accumulation (hydrops)
- Swelling of the labyrinthine system

Meniere's Disease

- Tinnitus
- Sensorineural hearing loss
  - Weber louder normal ear
  - Rinne: AC>BC
- Vertigo

Meniere's Disease

- Treatment
  - Avoid high salt – decrease swelling
  - Avoid caffeine, nicotine–vasoconstrictors, ↓flow from inner ear
  - Diuretics

Thalamus, Hypothalamus, Limbic System

Jason Ryan, MD, MPH

Subcortical Structures

- Thalamus
- Hypothalamus

- Basal Ganglia
  - Substantia Nigra
  - Subthalamic nucleus
  - Putamen
  - Caudate nucleus
  - Globus pallidus

Coronal Section

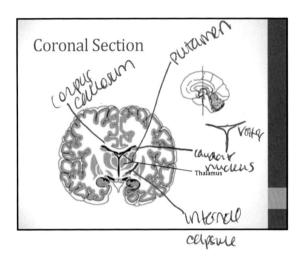

corpus callosum

Putamen

ventricle

caudate nucleus

Thalamus

internal capsule

Axial Section

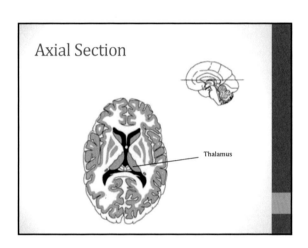

Thalamus

Thalamus

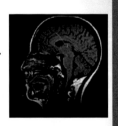

- "Gateway to the cortex"
- Greek word: "Inner chamber"
- Sits on top of brainstem
- Symmetrical – two halves
- Sensory relay → cortex
  - Except olfaction
- Consciousness
- Sleep
- Alertness

Thalamic Nuclei

- Many, many thalamic nuclei
- Most named by location
  - Anterior, posterior, ventral, medial
- Five nuclei worth knowing
  - Ventral posterorlateral (VPL)
  - Ventral posteromedial (VPM)
  - Lateral geniculate nucleus (LGN)
  - Medial geniculate nucleus (MGN)
  - Ventral lateral (VL)

Thalamic Nuclei

Nucleus	Info	Input	Output
VPL	All Sensory – pain, temp, touch, prop, vibration	Spinthalamic, Post column-medial leminiscus	Somatosensory cortex
VPM	Sensory face and taste	Trigeminal and gustatory	Somatosensory cortex
LGN	Vision	CN II	Calcarine Sulcus
MGN	Hearing	Superior olive and inferior colliculus of tectum	Temp Lobe – Auditory Cortex
VL	Motor	Basal ganglia	Motor Cortex

Thalamic Syndrome

- Usually a lacunar stroke
- Contralateral sensory loss
  - Face, arms, legs
  - All sensory modalities
- Resolution can lead to long term chronic pain
  - Contralateral side
  - Sensory exam normal
  - Severe pain in paroxysms or exacerbated by touch

Hypothalamus

- Found below thalamus
- Like thalamus, many nuclei with different functions

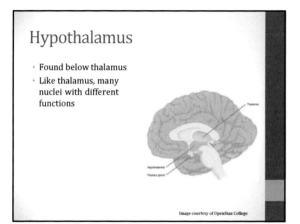

Image courtesy of OpenStax College

Hypothalamic Functions

- Autonomic control
  - Excites sympathetic/parasympathetic system
- Temperature regulation
- Water balance
- Pituitary control

Hypothalamic Areas

Area	Functions	Lesion
Lateral	Hunger	Anorexia Failure to thrive in infants
Ventromedial	Satiety	Hyperphagia, obesity
Anterior	Cooling	Hyperthermia
Posterior	Heating	Inability to thermoregulate
Suprachiasmatic nucleus	Circadian rhythm	--

Fever

- Triggered by pyrogens, inflammatory proteins
- IL-1, IL-6, and TNF enter brain
- Stimulate prostaglandin E2 synthesis
  - Via arachidonic acid pathway
  - Mediated by PLA2, COX-2, and prostaglandin E2 synthase
- Increases anterior hypothalamus set point
- Temp >42C = hyperpyrexia
- May cause permanent brain damage
  - Facilitate heat loss: cooling blankets, fans
  - Lower set point: NSAIDs, tylenol (block PGE2 synthesis)

Hormones

- Hypothalamus releases multiple hormones to stimulate release of other hormones from anterior pituitary
- TRH → TSH
- CRH → ACTH
- GHRH → Growth Hormone (GH)
- GNRH → FSH, LH

Hormones

- Some HT substances shut down hormone release
  - Dopamine (prolactin inhibiting hormone)→ ↓Prolactin
  - Somatostatin (GHRH inhibiting hormone)→ ↓ GH
- Prolactin feedback → ↓ GnRH

Hormones

- ADH and Oxytocin synthesized by HT
- Supraoptic nucleus → ADH
- Paraventricular nucleus → Oxytocin
- Both stored/released by posterior pituitary
  - ** Post. Pituitary also called neurohypophysis
  - ** Ant. Pituitary also called adenohypophysis
- Loss of ADH → Diabetes Insipidus
  - Polyuria, polydipsia, dilute urine

Leptin

- Hormone secreted by adipocytes
- Involved in food intake
- Regulation of homeostasis
- Lateral HT (hunger) → inhibited by Leptin
- Ventromedial (satiety) → stimulated by Leptin

Craniopharyngioma

- Rare tumor from Rathke's pouch
- Pressure on optic chiasm
  - Bitemporal hemianopia
- Pressure on hypothalamus
- Hypothalamic syndrome

Hypothalamic Syndrome

- Diabetes insipidus (loss of ADH)
- Fatigue (loss of CRH → low cortisol)
- Obesity
- Loss of temperature regulation

Limbic System

- Emotion
- Long-term memory
- Smell
- Behavior modulation
- Autonomic nervous system function

Limbic System
Key Components

- Cingulate gyrus
- Hippocampus
- Fornix
- Amygdala
- Mammillary bodies

Image courtesy of Anant Rathi

Kluver-Bucy Syndrome

- Damage to bilateral amygdala (temporal lobes)
- Hyperphagia - Weight gain
- Hyperorality - tendency to examine with mouth
- Inappropriate Sexual Behavior
  - Atypical sexual behavior, mounting inanimate objects
- Visual Agnosia
  - Inability to recognize visually presented objects
- Rare complication of HSV1 encephalitis

Hippocampus Lesion

- Anterograde amnesia
- Cannot make new memories
- Very sensitive to hypoxic damage
- Infarction:
  - Hippocampal branches PCA
  - Anterior choroidal arteries

Wernicke-Korsakoff Syndrome

- Wernicke: Acute encephalopathy
- Korsakoff: Chronic neurologic condition
  - Usually a consequence of Wernicke
- Both associated with: Thiamine
  - Thiamine (B1) deficiency
  - Alcoholism
- Atrophy of mammillary bodies common finding
  - 80% for both conditions
- Associated with damage to thalamic nuclei

Wernicke-Korsakoff Syndrome

- Triad Wernicke:
  - Visual disturbances/nystagmus
  - Gait ataxia
  - Confusion
  - Often reversible with thiamine
- Korsakoff: Amnesia
  - Recent memory affected more than remote
  - Can't form new memories
  - Confabulation: Can't remember so make things up
  - Lack of interest or concern
  - Personality changes
  - Usually permanent

Wernicke-Korsakoff Syndrome

- Wernicke precipitated by glucose without thiamine
  - Thiamine co-factor glucose metabolism
  - Glucose will worsen thiamine deficiency
- Banana bag
  - IV infusion to alcoholics
  - Thiamine, folic acid, and magnesium sulfate

Cerebellum

Jason Ryan, MD, MPH

Cerebellum

- "Little brain"
- Posture/balance
- Muscle tone
- Coordinates movement

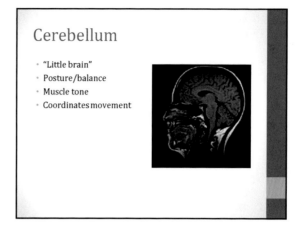

Anatomy

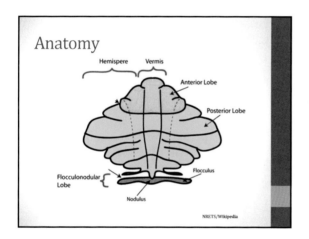

NRETS/Wikipedia

Cerebellar Peduncles
In and Out Pathways

- Inferior cerebellar peduncle
- Middle cerebellar peduncle
- Superior cerebellar peduncle

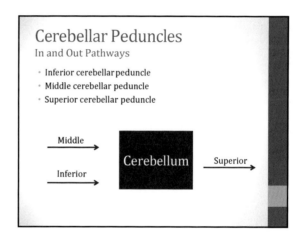

Inferior Cerebellar Peduncle

- Major pathway INTO cerebellum from spine
- Numerous inputs:
  - Spinocerebellar tract
  - Cuneocerebellar tract
  - Olivocerebellar tract
  - Vestibulocerebellar tract
- Ipsilateral spinal cord information: proprioception

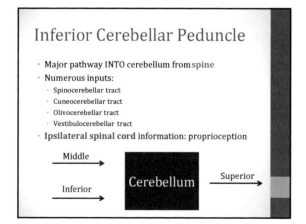

Middle Cerebellar Peduncle

- Pontocerebellar tract fibers
- Fibers from contralateral pons

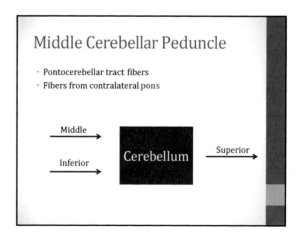

Climbing and Mossy Fibers

- Two types of axons that enter cerebellum
- Climbing fibers: arise from inferior olivary nucleus
- Mossy fibers: all other cerebellar inputs
- Synapse on Purkinje cells and deep nuclei

Superior Cerebellar Peduncle

- Major pathway OUT of cerebellum
- Axons from deep cerebellar nuclei
- All outputs originate from deep nuclei
- Fibers to red nucleus and thalamus

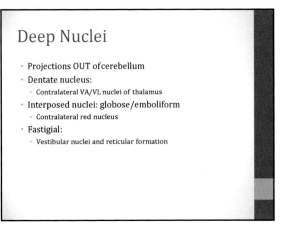

Purkinje Cells

- Cerebellar neurons
- Receive numerous inputs
- Project to deep nuclei
- Inhibitory
- Release GABA

Wikipedia/Public Domain

Deep Nuclei

- Projections OUT of cerebellum
- Dentate nucleus:
  - Contralateral VA/VL nuclei of thalamus
- Interposed nuclei: globose/emboliform
  - Contralateral red nucleus
- Fastigial:
  - Vestibular nuclei and reticular formation

Deep Nuclei

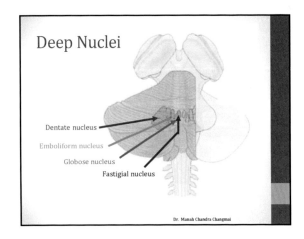

Dentate nucleus
Emboliform nucleus
Globose nucleus
Fastigial nucleus

Dr. Manah Chandra Changmai

Cerebellar Circuitry

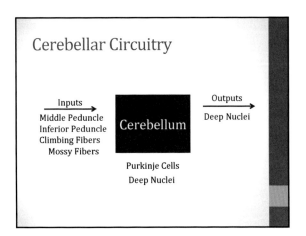

Inputs
Middle Peduncle
Inferior Peduncle
Climbing Fibers
Mossy Fibers

Cerebellum

Outputs
Deep Nuclei

Purkinje Cells
Deep Nuclei

Cerebellum Control

- In general, cerebellum controls IPSILATERAL side
- Cerebellar fibers → contralateral cortex
- Contralateral cortex → contralateral arm/leg
- Crosses twice
- Also right proprioception → right cerebellum
- Result:
  - Left cerebellar lesion → left symptoms
  - Right cerebellar lesion → right symptoms

Clinical Disease

- Lateral lesions
  - Cerebellar hemispheres
  - Dentate nucleus
  - Affect extremities
- Midline lesions
  - Vermis
  - Emboliform, globus and fastigial nuclei
  - Floculonodular lobe
  - Affect trunk

Lateral Lesions

- Extremities
- Direction, force, speed, and amplitude of movements
- Lesions:
  - Dysmetria
  - Intention tremor
- Fall toward injured side

Central Lesions

- Affect trunk/midline
- Central (vermis)
  - Truncal ataxia
  - Can't stand independently
  - Falls over when sitting
- Flocculonodular lobe
  - Connects to vestibular nuclei
  - Lesions: nystagmus, vertigo

Cerebellar Ataxia

- Loss of balance
- Classically a "wide-based" gait

Romberg Test

- Test for sensory (not cerebellar) ataxia
- Loss of proprioception: compensate through vision
- Feet together, eyes closed
- Positive test: patients will lose balance or fall
- If test positive: ataxia is SENSORY
- Cerebellar ataxia occurs even with eyes open

Other Cerebellar Symptoms

- Hypotonia
  - Loss of muscle resistance to passive manipulation
  - Loose-jointed, floppy joints
- Scanning speech
  - Irregular speech
  - "How are you doing?"
  - "How...are...you...do...ing"
- Dyssynergia

Dyssynergia
Loss of coordinated activity

- Dysmetria
  - Loss of movement coordination
  - Under or over-shoot intended position of hand
- Intention tremor
  - Can't get hand to target
  - Contrast with resting tremor (Parkinson's)
- Dysdiadochokinesia
  - Can't make movements exhibiting a rapid change of motion
  - Can't flip hand in palm

Other Cerebellar Symptoms

- Nystagmus
  - Up/down beat (vertical)
  - Gaze-evoked
- Nausea/vomiting
- Vertigo

Cerebellar Strokes

- SCA, AICA, PICA
- Often has other brainstem stroke signs/symptoms

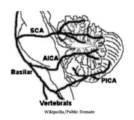

Wikipedia/Public Domain

Hereditary Ataxias

- Numerous hereditary disorders
- Motor incoordination related to cerebellum
- Ataxia Telangiectasia
- Friedreich's Ataxia

Ataxia Telangiectasia

- Autosomal recessive
- Cerebellar atrophy
  - Ataxia in 1st year of life
- Telangiectasias
  - Dilation of capillary vessels on skin
  - Ears, nose, face, and neck
- Repeated sinus/respiratory infections
  - Severe immunodeficiency
- High risk of cancer

Ataxia Telangiectasia
Clinical Features

- Most children healthy for first year
- Begin walking at normal age but slow development
- Progressive motor coordination problems
- By 10 years old, most in wheelchairs
- Other symptoms
  - Recurrent sinus/respiratory infections
  - Telangiectasias
- **High risk of cancer**

Ataxia Telangiectasia

- Cause: **DNA hypersensitivity to ionizing radiation**
- Defective ATM gene on chromosome 11
  - Ataxia Telangiectasia Mutated gene
  - Repairs double stranded DNA breaks
  - Nonhomologous end-joining (NHEJ)
- Mutation: Failure to repair DNA mutations

Nonhomologous end-joining
NHEJ

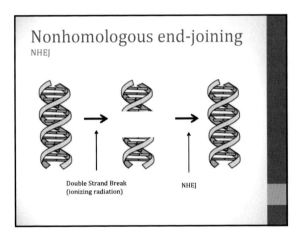

Double Strand Break   NHEJ
(ionizing radiation)

Ataxia Telangiectasia
Lab Abnormalities

- ↑AFP
  - Often elevated in pregnant women
  - Also elevated in ataxia telangiectasia
  - Most consistent lab finding
- Dysgammaglobulinemia
  - Low or absent IgA

Friedreich's Ataxia

- Autosomal recessive
- Mutation of **frataxin gene** chromosome 9
  - Needed for normal mitochondrial function
  - Increased number of trinucleotide (GAA) repeats present
  - More repeats = worse prognosis
  - Leads to decreased frataxin levels
- Frataxin: **mitochondrial protein**
  - High levels in brain, heart, and pancreas
  - Abnormal frataxin → mitochondrial dysfunction

Friedreich's Ataxia

- Begins in adolescence with progressive symptoms
- Cerebellar and spinal cord degeneration
- Degeneration of spinocerebellar tract
  - Ataxia, dysarthria
- Loss of spinal cord: dorsal columns
  - Position/vibration
- Loss of corticospinal tract
  - UMN weakness in lower extremity

Friedreich's Ataxia
Other Features

- Hypertrophic cardiomyopathy
- Diabetes
  - Insulin resistance and impaired insulin release
  - Beta cell dysfunction

Friedreich's Ataxia
Other Features

- Kyphoscoliosis
- Foot abnormalities (pes cavus)
  - High arch of foot; does not flatten with weight bearing
  - Seen in other neuromuscular diseases (Charcot-Marie-Tooth)

Axelrod FB, Gold-von Simson G.

Benefros/Wikipedia

Other Cerebellar Disorders

- Tumors
  - Pilocytic astrocytoma
  - Medulloblastoma
  - Ependymoma
- Congenital disease
  - Dandy Walker malformation
  - Chiari malformations

Basal Ganglia

Jason Ryan, MD, MPH

Basal Ganglia

- Substantia Nigra
- Subthalamic nucleus
- Putamen
- Caudate nucleus
- Globus pallidus

Basal Ganglia

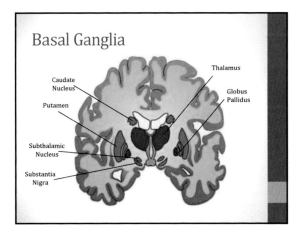

Basal Ganglia Terms

- Striatum = Putamen + Caudate
  - Also called striate nucleus
  - Putamen/Caudate divided by internal capsule
  - Major INPUT from cortex
- Lentiform Nucleus = Putamen + Globus Palidus

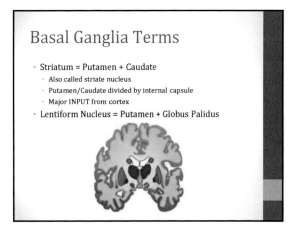

Function

- Modifies voluntary movements
- Receives cortex input
- Provides feedback to cortex to either
  - #1: Stimulate motor activity
  - #2: Inhibit motor activity
- Combination stim/inhibition → complex movements

Movement Execution

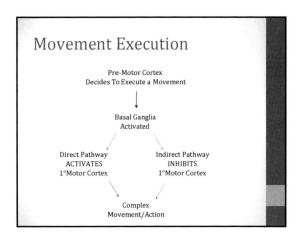

Basal Ganglia Connections

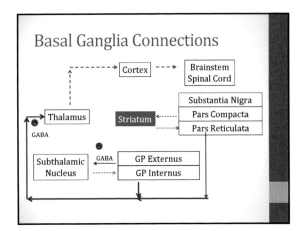

To Stimulate Movement
Direct Pathway

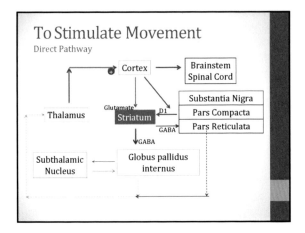

To Inhibit Movement
Indirect Pathway

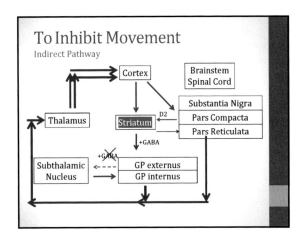

Key Points

- Direct pathway
  - Goal is to create movement
  - Striatum inhibits (GABA) GPi and Pars Reticulata
  - GPi and Pars STOP inhibiting Thalamus
  - Thalamus free to activate cortex
- Modifier: SN pars compacta modifies striatum via D1

Key Points

- Indirect pathway
  - Goal is to further inhibit movement
  - Striatum inhibits GPe (GABA)
  - GPe stops inhibiting Subthalamic nucleus
  - Subthalamic nucleus stimulates GPi
  - GPi further inhibits thalamus
- Modifier: SN pars compacta modifies striatum via D2

Pars Compacta

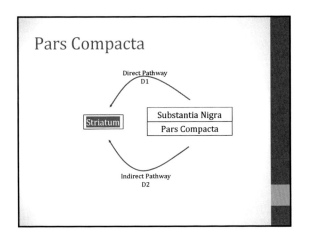

Movement Disorders

- Parkinson's disease
- Huntington's Disease
- Hemiballism
- Wilson's Disease
- All result from damage to part of basal ganglia

Basal Ganglia Connections

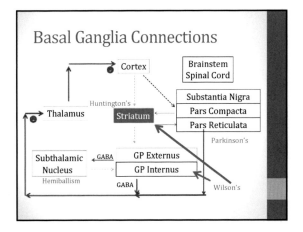

Ventricles and Sinuses

Jason Ryan, MD, MPH

CNS Ventricles

- Four structures that contain CSF in brain
  - Two lateral ventricles
  - 3rd ventricle
  - 4th ventricle
- Continuous with central canal of spinal cord

Ventricles

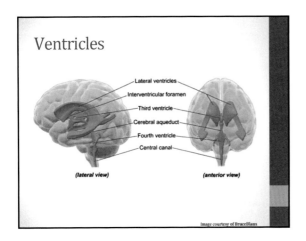

Lateral ventricles
Interventricular foramen
Third ventricle
Cerebral aqueduct
Fourth ventricle
Central canal

(lateral view)   (anterior view)

Image courtesy of BruceBlaus

Ventricles

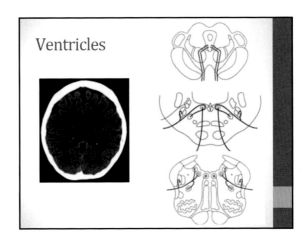

Cerebrospinal Fluid

- Clear, colorless fluid
- Acts as cushion for brain
  - Mechanical protection
  - Shock absorber
- Also circulates nutrients removes waste

CSF Production

- Production
  - Ependymal cells of choroid plexus (ventricles)
- Absorption
  - Arachnoid villi
- CSF drained to superior sagittal sinus
  - Then to venous system

Choroid Plexus Cysts

- Can be detected by ultrasound in utero
- A normal finding but associated with chromosome abnormalities

Hydrocephalus

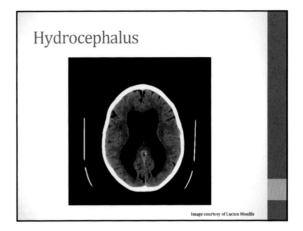

Image courtesy of Lucien Monfils

Hydrocephalus

- Dilation of ventricles
- Excessive accumulation of CSF
- Communicating
  - Ventricles CAN communicate
  - CSF not being absorbed
- Non-communicating
  - There is a blockage to flow
  - Ventricles CAN'T communicate

Communicating Hydrocephalus

- ↓ CSF absorption by arachnoid, ↑ ICP
- Headache
- Key sign: papilledema
- CT Hallmark: Dilation ALL ventricles
- Often occurs from scarring after meningitis
- Can cause herniation
- Key clinical scenario
  - Prior meningitis
  - Headache
  - Papilledema on eye exam
  - Enlarged ventricles on CT scan

Non-Communicating Hydrocephalus

- Structural blockage of CSF flow within ventricles
- Often congenital
- Many etiologies
- Three worth knowing:
  - Aqueductal stenosis
  - Chiari Malformations
  - Dandy Walker malformation

Aqueductal Stenosis

- Stenosis of cerebral aqueduct
- Blocked drainage from 3rd to 4th ventricle
- Congenital narrowing
  - X-linked (boys)
- Inflammation due to intrauterine infection
  - Rubella, CMV, toxo, syphilis
- Presentation: Enlarging head circumference

Chiari II Malformation

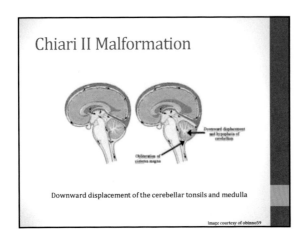

Downward displacement of the cerebellar tonsils and medulla

Image courtesy of obinno59

Myelomeningocele
(Spina Bifida)

- Type of neural tube defect
- Failure of spine and meninges to close around cord
- Myelomeningocele: cord/meninges outside spine
- Almost always has Chiari II malformation
- Hydrocephalus major cause morbidity
- Obstruction 4th ventricular outflow

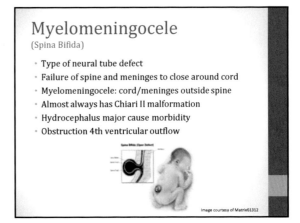

Image courtesy of Matrix61312

Dandy Walker Malformation

- Developmental anomaly of the fourth ventricle
- Hypoplasia or agenesis of cerebellar vermis
- Cysts of 4th ventricle → hydrocephalus
- Massive 4th ventricle, small cerebellum
- Many, many associated symptoms/conditions
- Affected children
  - Hydrocephalus (macrocephaly)
  - Delayed development
  - Motor dysfunction (crawling, walking)

Dandy Walker Malformation

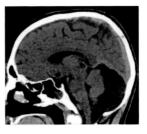

Pseudotumor Cerebri

- Idiopathic intracranial hypertension
- ↑ICP in absence of tumor or other cause
- Intractable, disabling headaches
- Papilledema, visual loss
- Pulsatile tinnitus
  - Rushing water or wind sound
  - Transmission of vascular pulsations
- Classic patient: overweight woman, childbearing age
- Diagnosis: spinal tap (measure pressure)
- Medical treatment: acetazolamide

Normal Pressure Hydrocephalus (NPH)

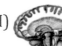

- Enlarged ventricles on imaging
- Compression of corona radiata
- Normal opening pressure on LP
- Suspected mechanism: Impaired absorption CSF
- Classic triad:
  - Urinary incontinence, gait disturbance, dementia
  - Wet, wobbly, and wacky
- Treatment: Ventriculoperitoneal(VP) Shunt
  - Drains CSF to abdomen

66

Hydrocephalus ex Vacuo

- Ventricular enlargement that:
  - Occurs with age
  - As cortex atrophies (Alzheimer's, Pick, HIV)
- Brain shrinkage
- Usually after age 60
- Increase size of ventricles
  - IN PROPORTION to increase size of sulci
- If out of proportion: hydrocephalus

Dural Sinuses

- Large venous channels
- Travel through dura
- Drain blood from cerebral veins
- Receive CSF from arachnoid granulations
- Empty into internal jugular vein

Dural Sinuses

Some Key Sinuses

- Sagittal – Superior sagittal receives CSF
- Cavernous

Cavernous Sinus

- Large collection veins
- Bilateral
- Between temporal/sphenoid bones
- Collects blood eye/cortex
- Drains into internal jugular vein
- Many nerves:
  - CN III, IV, V1, V2 , VI, sympathetic fibers
  - All traveling to orbit
- Also portion of internal carotid artery

Cavernous Sinus Syndrome

- Compression by tumor, thrombus, fistula
- Infections of face, nose, orbits, tonsils, and soft palate can spread to cavernous sinus (septic thrombosis)
- Internal carotid travels THROUGH venous structure
  - Rupture carotid → fistula
- Symptoms
  - Headache
  - Swollen eyes
  - Impairment of ocular motor nerves
  - Horner's syndrome
  - Sensory loss 1st/2nd divisions trigeminal nerve

AV Malformations

- Artery to vein connection → no capillary bed
- Enlarge over time
- Commonly result in Vein of Galen enlargement
- Usually occur in utero
- May be asymptomatic until adolescence/adulthood
- Cause headaches and seizures

AV Malformations

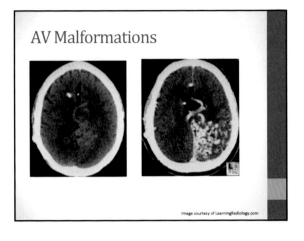

Image courtesy of LearningRadiology.com

Cerebral and Lacunar Strokes

Jason Ryan, MD, MPH

Etiology

- Ischemic (80%)
  - Insufficient blood flow
  - Thrombosis, embolism, hypoperfusion
  - Symptom onset over hours
- Hemorrhagic (20%)
  - Brain bleeding
  - Sudden onset
- Best first test: Non-contrast CT of head

CNS Blood Supply

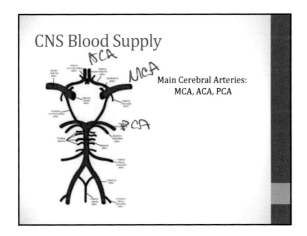

Main Cerebral Arteries:
MCA, ACA, PCA

Homunculus

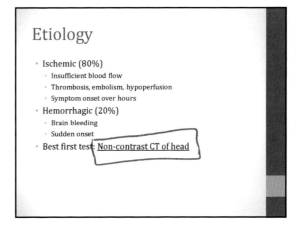

MCA: Upper limb, face
ACA: Lower limb
PCA: Vision

Image courtesy of Wikipiedia and OpenStax College

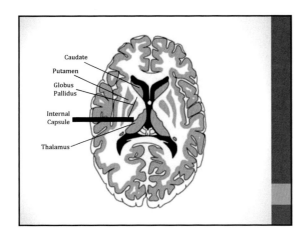

Caudate
Putamen
Globus Pallidus
Internal Capsule
Thalamus

MCA Stroke

- A 75-year-old man presents with recent onset loss of movement of his right arm. The right side of his face also droops and there is drooling from the corner of his mouth on the right side. He has difficulty speaking.

MCA Stroke

- Most common site of stroke
- Contralateral motor/sensory sx
- Arm>leg, face
- Spastic (UMN) paralysis
- If left sided
  - Aphasia
  - Speech center is left sided most patients
- If right (nondominant) side
  - Hemineglect

Lower Facial Droop

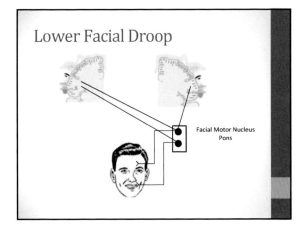

Facial Motor Nucleus
Pons

Lower Facial Droop

- Upper face: Dual UMN supply; right & left
- Lower face: Single UMN supply
  - Contralateral Motor Cortex
  - Fibers run in corticobulbar tract
- MCA stroke damage → UMN damage
  - Upper face intact (dual supply)
  - Lower face affected

CT Head

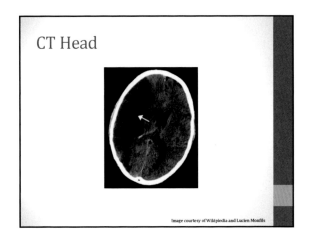

Image courtesy of Wikipiedia and Lucien Monfils

ACA Stroke

- A 75-year-old man presents with acute loss of ability to move his right hip and leg. On exam, he has decreased sensation to pinprick and vibration of his right leg.

Anterior Cerebral Artery (ACA)

- Left ACA stroke
- Leg>Arm
- Second most common stroke site
- Medial cortex (midline portion)
- Leg-foot area (motor and sensory)

PCA Stroke

- An 80-year-old man presents with acute <u>visual loss</u>. He reports difficulty seeing objects on his right side. His wife said he also reports seeing people who are not in the room. On exam, there are <u>no motor or sensory deficits</u>. Visual fields are shown below (black = no vision).

PCA Stroke

- Posterior portion of brain
- Visual cortex
- Visual hallucinations
- Visual agnosia (seeing things but can't recognize)
- Contralateral hemianopia with macular sparing

Homonymous Hemianopsia

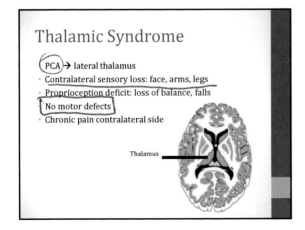

Left PCA Stroke Left
Optic Tract Lesion
Right visual loss

Right PCA Stroke Right
Optic Tract Lesion Left
visual loss

Macular Sparing

- Macula: central, high-resolution vision (reading)
- Dual blood supply: MCA and PCA
- PCA strokes often spare the macula

Thalamic Syndrome

- PCA → lateral thalamus
- Contralateral sensory loss: face, arms, legs
- Proprioception deficit: loss of balance, falls
- No motor defects
- Chronic pain contralateral side

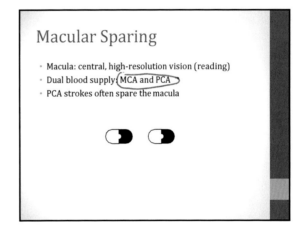

Thalamus

Hypoxic Encephalopathy

- Loss of CNS blood flow
- Loss of consciousness <10sec
- Permanent damage <4min
  - Neurons: No glycogen storage!
- Coma, vegetative states common
- Causes:
  - Shock
  - Anemia
  - Repeated hypoglycemia

Hypoxic Encephalopathy

- Hippocampus (pyramidal cells) first area damaged
- Cerebellum (Purkinje cells) also highly susceptible

Watershed Area Infarct

- Most distal branches of major arteries vulnerable
  - "Watershed infract"
- Borders between MCA/ACA/PCA
- Classic scenario: CNS damage after massive MI

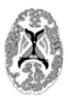

Watershed Area

- Weakness of the shoulders and thighs
- Sparing of the face, hands, and feet
- Bilateral symptoms
- A "man-in-a-barrel"

Lacunar Strokes

- Anatomically small strokes associated with HTN
- Stroke resolves and leaves lacunae in brain
  - Lacunae = Latin for "empty space"
- May not show initial CT
- Also associated with DM, smoking

Lacunar Strokes

- Noncortical infarcts
- Different from ACA, MCA, PCA
- Lack "cortical signs"
  - Aphasia, agnosia, or hemianopsia

Common Locations

- Internal capsule
- Thalamus
- Basal ganglia
- Pons

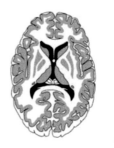

Vessels

handwritten note: internal capsule, Basal ganglia

- Lenticulostriate branches (MCA)
- Anterior choroidal artery (ICA)
- Recurrent artery of Heubner (ACA)
- Thalamoperforate branch (PCA)
- Paramedian branches (basilar artery)

Lacunar Strokes

- Substrate: arteriolar sclerosis (HTN)
- Proposed causes:
  - Lipohyalinosis: small vessel destruction, necrosis
  - Microatheroma: macrophages in vessel

Lacunar Strokes

Subtype	Symptoms	Other Details
Pure Motor	Paralysis of face, arm and leg on one side	Posterior limb internal Capsule
Pure Sensory	Numbness, sensory loss one side of body: Face, arm, and leg	VPL Thalamus
Sensorimotor	Paralysis & sensory loss	Thalamus, internal capsule, caudate and putamen, and pons
Ataxic Hemiparesis	Weakness, dysarthria, ataxia out of proportion to weakness	Base pons, internal capsule
Dysarthria-Clumsy Hand Syndrome	Dysarthria and clumsiness (weakness) of the hand	Pons, internal capsule

Hemiballism

- Wild, flinging movements of extremities (ballistic)
- Damage to subthalamic nucleus
- Seen in rare subtypes of lacunar strokes

Classic Lacunar Stroke

- Patient with uncontrolled hypertension
- Symptoms consistent with 1 of 5 lacunar subtypes
  - Pure motor (legs=arms; internal capsule)
  - Pure sensory (thalamus)
- Negative initial head CT

73

Vertebral Basilar Stroke Syndromes

Jason Ryan, MD, MPH

Vertebral Artery Anatomy

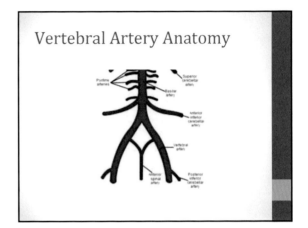

Brainstem Blood Supply

Lateral   Medial

PCA

AICA

    Basilar

PICA

    ASA

3	Midbrain
4	
6 5,7,8	Pons
12 9,10,11	Medulla

SCA Stroke

- Rarest of all cerebellar (AICA, PICA) strokes
- Mostly cerebellar symptoms
- Ipsilateral cerebellar ataxias
- Nausea and vomiting

Basilar Artery Stroke

- Locked-in Syndrome
- Ventral pontine syndrome
- Loss of corticospinal and corticobulbar tracts
- Bilateral paralysis (quadrapalegia)
- Patient can blink (upper brainstem intact)
- Contrast with vegetative state
  - Motor function intact
  - Cortical dysfunction

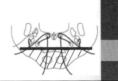

Central Pontine Myelinolysis
"Osmotic demeyelination syndrome"

- Demyelination of central pontine axons
- Lesion at base of pons
- Loss of corticospinal and corticobulbar tracts
- Associated with overly rapid correction ↓Na
- Quadriplegia
- Can be similar to locked-in syndrome

Top of the Basilar Syndrome

- Very rare
- Occlusion of upper basilar artery (usually embolic)
- Changes in the level of consciousness (coma)
- Visual symptoms: hallucinations, blindness
- Eye problems:
  - 3rd nerve palsy
  - Loss of vertical gaze
  - Problems with convergence
- Usually no significant motor loss

Key VB Stroke Syndromes

- AICA
- PICA
- ASA

AICA Stroke

- Lateral pontine syndrome
- Vestibular nuclei: nystagmus, vertigo, N/V
- Spinothalamic tract: Contralateral pain/temp
- Spinal V nucleus: ipsilateral face pain/temp
- Sympathetic tract: Horner's syndrome
- Facial nucleus:
  - Ipsilateral facial droop
  - Loss corneal reflex
- Cochlear nuclei
  - Deafness
- Taste on anterior tongue (VII)

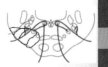

Horner's Syndrome

- Compression/disruption sympathetic ganglia
- Hypothalamus → T1 → Face/eyes
- Lesion anywhere along pathway = Horner's
- Miosis, ptosis, and anhidrosis
- Small/constricted pupil (miosis)
  - Unequal pupils
  - Affected side smaller
- Drooping eyelid (ptosis)
- No sweat (anhidrosis)

PICA Stroke

- Lateral medullary (Wallenberg's) syndrome
- Vestibular nuclei: Nystagmus, vertigo, N/V
- Sympathetic tract: Horner's syndrome
- Spinothalamic tract: Contralateral pain/temp
- Spinal V nucleus: ipsilateral face pain/temp
- Nucleus ambiguus (IX, X)
  - Hoarseness, dysphagia, ↓gag reflex

ASA Stroke

- Midline structures damaged
- Can affect medulla or spinal cord

ASA Stroke
Level of Spinal Cord

- Anterior spinal artery syndrome
- ASA supplies anterior 2/3 of spinal cord
- Loss of all but posterior columns
- Only vibration, proprioception intact
- Paralysis below lesion

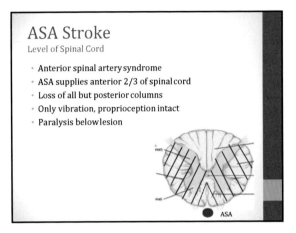

ASA

ASA Stroke
Level of Medulla

- Medial medullary syndrome
- Corticospinal, medial lemniscus, CN 12
- Contralateral Hemiparesis
- Contralateral loss of proprioception/vibration
- Flaccid paralysis tongue
  - Deviation to side of lesion

Key VB Stroke Syndromes

Vessel	Area	Key Findings
AICA	Lateral pons	Facial droop, hearing loss
PICA	Lateral medulla	Dysphagia, hoarseness
ASA	Medial medulla	Contralateral motor, tongue deviation
	Anterior spine	Bilateral motor, pain, temp; sparing vibratrion/proprio

Cerebral Aneurysms

Jason Ryan, MD, MPH

Aneurysms

- Weak vessel wall
- Abnormal dilation

Aneurysms

- Saccular or Berry
  - More common type
- Charcot-Bouchard aneurysms
  - Microaneurysm
  - Cause of hemorrhagic stroke in HTN
  - Severe HTN
  - Similar: lacunar strokes

Berry Aneurysms Associations

- ADPKD
- Ehlers-Danlos
- Aortic coarctation
- Older age
- Hypertension
- Smoking
- African Americans

Aneurysm Rupture

- Subarachnoid hemorrhage (berry)
  - Bleeding into CSF space
  - Neuro symptoms rare → mostly headache
- Hemorrhagic stroke (micro)
  - Symptoms based on site of bleeding

Subarachnoid Hemorrhage

- Bleeding into space b/w arachnoid & pia mater

tracks along space between lobs

Image courtesy of James Heilman, MD

Subarachnoid Hemorrhage

- "Worst headache of my life"
- Sudden onset symptoms
- Fever, nuchal rigidity common
- CT scan usually diagnostic
- Xanthochromia on spinal tap — *yellow discoloration*
- No focal deficits!

Subarachnoid Hemorrhage

- Treat with clipping or endovascular coiling
- Re-bleeding common
- Vasospasm
  - Triggered by blood
  - Worsening neuro symptoms
  - Days after initial bleed
- Nimodipine (calcium-channel blocker)
  - Improves outcome
  - Unclear mechanism
  - May prevent vasospasm

Berry Aneurysm Sites

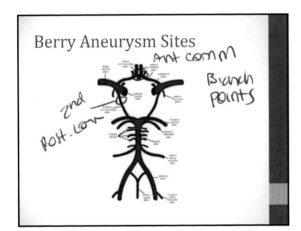

Ant comm
Branch points
2nd
Post. comm

AComm Aneurysm

- Headache
- Visual field defects

Bitemporal Hemianopsia
Optic Chiasm Compression
Pituitary Tumor/Aneurysm

PComm Aneurysm

- Unilateral headache, eye pain
- CN III palsy
  - Eye: "down and out"
  - Ptosis
  - Pupil dilation – nonreactive to light

Pupil Sparing

- Is pupil normal (not dilated)?
- If yes, pupil is spared → lesion not aneurysm
- Pupillary constrictors easily compressed in subarachnoid space
- If pupil is "spared"
  - Palsy often associated with DM
  - Ischemic neuropathy of CN III (small vessel disease)
  - Sometimes painful
  - Spontaneously resolves
- "Rule of the pupil"

Charcot-Bouchard Aneurysms

- Micro-aneurysms
- Small branches lenticulo-striate arteries
- Basal ganglia, thalamus
- Possible origin of hypertensive ICH

Intracranial Bleeding

Jason Ryan, MD, MPH

Raised Intracranial Pressure
ICP

- Mass lesions (tumors)
- Cerebral edema (large stroke, severe trauma)

- Obstruction of venous outflow (thrombosis)
- Idiopathic intracranial hypertension
  - Pseudotumor cerebri

Increased Intracranial Pressure
General symptoms

- Headache (pain fibers CN V in dura)
- Depressed consciousness
  - Pressure on midbrain reticular formation
- Vomiting

Papilledema

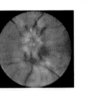
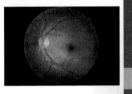

- Optic disc swelling
- Due to ↑ICP
  - i.e. mass effect
- Also seen in severe HTN
- Usually bilateral
- Blurred margins optic disc on fundoscopy

Images courtesy of Warfieldian and OptometrusPrime

Cushing's Triad

- Hypertension
- Bradycardia
- Irregular respiration

Posturing

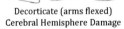

Decorticate (arms flexed)
Cerebral Hemisphere Damage

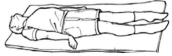

Decerebrate (arms extended)
Brainstem Damage

Image courtesy of Djsilverspoon

Glasgow Coma Scale

- Three tests: eye, verbal and motor
- GCS score: 3 to 15
- Eye (1-4 points)
  - Does not open, opens to painful stimuli, opens to voice, opens spontaneously
- Verbal (1-5 points)
  - No sound, incomprehensible sounds, inappropriate words, confused, oriented
- Motor (1-6 points)
  - No movements, decerebrate posturing, decorticate posturing, withdrawal to pain, localizes to pain, obeys commands

Herniation

- Expanding volume: blood, tumor
- Forces brain through weakest points

Where can displaced brain go?

- Subfalcine
  - Side to side
- Uncal
  - Side to bottom
  - Transtentorial
- Central
  - Diencephalon → midbrain
- Tonsillar
  - Cerebellum thru the "hole"

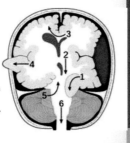

Image courtesy of aokianc.com

Subfalcine Herniation

- Cingulate gyrus
- Extends under falx
- Drags ipsilateral ACA with it
- ACA compression
- Contralateral leg paresis

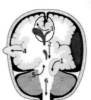

Uncal herniation

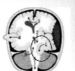

- Uncus = medial temporal lobe
- Across tentorium
- Midbrain compression

Uncal herniation

- Ipsilateral CNIII compression
  - Loss of parasympathetic innervation
  - Dilated ("blown") pupil
  - Lack of pupillary constriction to light
- Collapses ipsilateral posterior cerebral artery
  - Visual loss – cortical blindness
  - Homonymous hemianopsia
- Cerebral peduncle compression
  - Can be on side of lesion (contralateral paresis)
  - Can also be on opposite side (ipsilateral paresis)
    - Kernohan's notch
- Duret hemorrhage of pons and midbrain
  - Perforating branches basilar artery draining veins

Uncal herniation

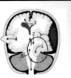

- Dilated pupil (side of lesion)
- Visual loss
- Hemiparesis or quadriparesis

Transtentorial Herniation

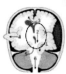

- Thalamus, hypothalamus, and medial parts of both temporal lobes forced through tentorium cerebelli
- Somnolence, LOC
- Initially: small, reactive pupils
- Later: nonreactive
- Posturing

Tonsillar Herniation

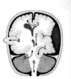

- Cerebellar tonsils herniate downward through the foramen magnum
- Most commonly caused by a posterior fossa mass lesion
- Compression of medulla results in depression centers for respiration and cardiac rhythm control
- Cardiorespiratory failure

Types of Intracranial Bleeds

- Epidural Hematoma
- Subdural Hematoma
- Subarachnoid Hemorrhage
- Hemorrhagic Stroke

The Meninges

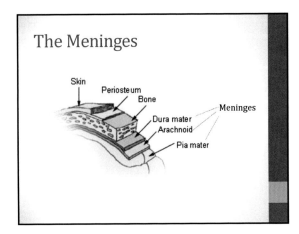

Epidural Hematoma

- Rupture of middle meningeal artery
  - Branch of maxillary artery
- Traumatic:
  - Often fracture of temporal bone
- Convex Shape on CT
- Dura attached sutures
  - Lesion cant cross suture lines

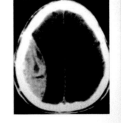

Image courtesy of Dryphi

Midline Shift

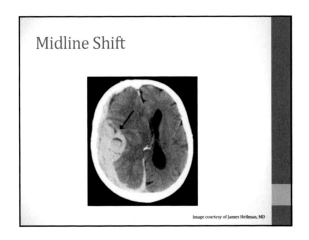

Maxillary Artery

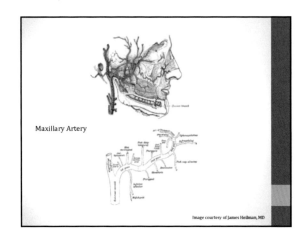

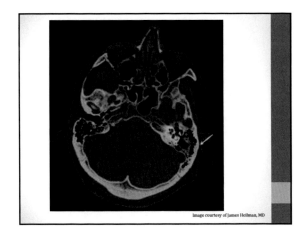

Epidural Hematoma
Symptoms

- General symptoms:
  - Headache, drowsiness, loss of consciousness
- Lucid interval

Subdural Hematoma

- Usually traumatic
- Rupture bridging veins
- Blood b/w dura and arachnoid space
- SLOW bleeding due to low pressure veins

Subdural Hematoma

- Crescent shaped bleed
- Crosses suture lines
- Limited by dural reflections
  - falx cerebri
  - tentorium
  - falx cerebelli

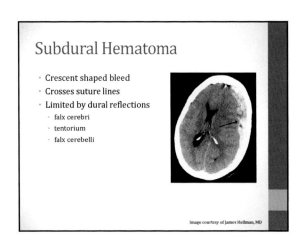

Subdural Hematoma

- Risk factors
  - Old age
  - Alcoholics
  - Blood thinners
- Brain atrophy increases space veins must cross
  - More vulnerable to rupture
- Classic history is confusion weeks after head injury
- Classic injury in shaken baby syndrome

Subarachnoid Hemorrhage

- Bleeding into space b/w arachnoid & pia mater

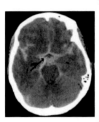

Image courtesy of James Heilman, MD

Subarachnoid Hemorrhage

- "Worst headache of my life"
- Sudden onset symptoms
- Fever, nuchal rigidity common
- CT scan usually diagnostic
- _Xanthochromia_ on spinal tap
- No focal deficits!

Subarachnoid Hemorrhage

- Usually from ruptured berry aneurysms
  - Most common site: anterior circle of Willis
  - Branch points of AComm artery
- AVMs
- Other associations:
  - Marfan syndrome
  - ADPKD
  - Ehlers-Danlos

Hemorrhagic Stroke
Intraparenchymal Bleed

- Often small arteries or arterioles
- HTN
- Anti-coagulation
- CNS malignancy
- Ischemic stroke followed by reperfusion

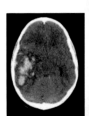

Image courtesy of OpenStax College

Sites of Bleed
Intraparenchymal Bleed

- Putamen (35%)
- Subcortex (30%)
- Cerebellum (16%)
- Thalamus (15%)
- Pons (5-12%)

Hemorrhage Stroke
Intraparenchymal Bleed

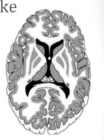

- Putamen stroke
- Contralateral hemiparesis (IC)
- Hemisensory loss (thalamus)
- Gaze deviation toward side of bleed (FEF)
- Watch for:
  - Left paralysis, sensory loss
  - Eyes deviated to right

Charcot-Bouchard Aneurysms

- Micro-aneurysms
- Small branches lenticulo-striate arteries
- Basal ganglia, thalamus
- Possible origin of hypertensive ICH

Cerebral Amyloid Angiopathy

- Recurrent hemorrhagic strokes
- Beta-amyloid deposits in artery walls
  - Weak, prone to rupture
- Typically lobar hemorrhages
  - Frontal, parietal, occipital
  - Usually smaller stokes
  - Contrast with HTN: Basal ganglia
- Watch for:
  - Elderly person
  - Recurrent hemorrhagic strokes

Intraventricular Hemorrhage

- Complication of premature birth
- Hemorrhage into lateral ventricle
- Usually first 5 days of life
- Sometimes asymptomatic
- LOC, hypotonia, loss of spontaneous movements
- Massive bleeds can cause seizures, coma

Intraventricular Hemorrhage

- Clot can obstruct the Foramen of Monro
  - Enlargement of lateral ventricles
  - Normal 3rd/4th ventricle
  - Treatment: Ventriculoperitoneal (VP)
- Germinal matrix problem
  - Highly vascular area near ventricles
  - Premature infants: poor autoregulation of blood flow here
  - In full term infants, this area has decreased vascularity

Treatment of TIA/Stroke

Jason Ryan, MD, MPH

Stroke

- Brain attack
- Patient appears "struck" down
- Sudden loss of neurological function
- Symptoms resolve <24 hrs = TIA
- Resolve >24hrs or persist = Stroke

Etiology

- Ischemic (80%)
  - Insufficient blood flow
  - Thrombosis, embolism, hypoperfusion
  - Symptom onset over hours
- Hemorrhagic (20%)
  - Brain bleeding
  - Sudden onset
- Best first test: Non-contrast CT of head
  - Provided patient is stable
- Diffusion weighted MRI is most accurate

Head CT

- Tells you ischemic versus hemorrhagic
- If ischemic must consider thrombolysis
- If hemorrhagic
  - Thrombolysis contraindicated
  - Reduce BP, reverse anti-coagulants, surgery
- NO benefit to heparin, warfarin, anti-platelets during acute stroke
  - Some role in prevention of recurrent stroke

Thrombolysis for Stroke

- 3-hour window of benefit for TPA (alteplase)
- Contraindications
  - Stroke or head trauma past 3 months
  - Arterial puncture in non-compressible site past week
  - Internal bleeding or trauma
  - BP>185/110
  - INR>1.7
  - Platelets <100k
  - Elevated PTT
  - Glucose <50mg/dL
  - ANY history of intracranial bleed

Post-Stroke Management

- Aspirin for prophylaxis
  - If allergic: clopidogrel
- EKG: Look for afib
  - Afib plus stroke = Warfarin or other AC
- Echocardiogram (source of embolism/PFO)
- Carotid ultrasound
  - Surgery considered if >70% stenosis

Stroke in Afib

- CHADs Score
  - CHF (1point)
  - HTN (1point)
  - Age >75yrs (1point)
  - Diabetes (1point)
  - Stroke (2point)
- Score >2 = Warfarin or other AC
- Score 0 -1 = Aspirin

Stroke

- CHADs VASC Score
  - CHF (1point)
  - HTN (1pont)
  - Diabetes (1point)
  - Stroke (2points)
  - Female (1point)
  - Age 65-75 (1point)
  - Age >75yrs (2points)
  - Vascular disease (1point)
- Score >2 = Warfarin or other AC
- Score 0 -1 = Aspirin

Anticoagulation

- Warfarin
  - Requires regular INR monitoring
  - Goal INR usually 2-3
- Rivaroxaban, Apixaban
  - Factor X inhibitors
- Dabigatran
  - Direct thrombin inhibitor
- Whether Afib persists or sinus rhythm restored anticoagulation MUST be addressed

Autonomic Nervous System

Jason Ryan, MD, MPH

Vocabulary

- Somatic
  - Greek: "Of the body"
  - Voluntary actions (muscles)
  - Movement, speech, etc.
- Autonomic
  - Auto = "self", nomos = "arrangement"
  - Involuntary actions
  - Salivation, vessel constriction, etc.
- Enteric – GI nervous system

Two Switch System

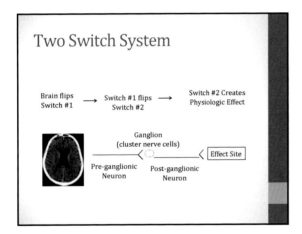

Brain flips Switch #1 → Switch #1 flips Switch #2 → Switch #2 Creates Physiologic Effect

Ganglion (cluster nerve cells)

Pre-ganglionic Neuron   Post-ganglionic Neuron   Effect Site

Synapses

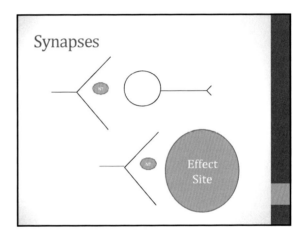

Effect Site

The Two Systems

- Sympathetic System
  - Fight or flight
- Parasympathetic System
  - Rest and digest

Sympathetic System
Major Actions

Activating Actions	Deactivating Actions
Eyes: dilates pupils	GI: ↓peristalsis
Lungs: dilates bronchioles	Skin: vasoconstriction
Heart: ↑ heart rate, contractility	↓saliva
Liver: Glycogen to glucose	↓tears
Kidneys: ↑ renin	Inhibit urination
↑sweat glands	Relaxes bladder
	Constricts urethra

Fight or Flight

88

Skin

- #1: Sympathetic effect: vasoconstriction
- #2: Exercise effects
  - Exercise → ↑ sympathetic → vasoconstriction
  - Exercise → ↑ temperature
  - Sensed by hypothalamus
  - Vasodilation
- #3: Heat dissipation aided by sweating
  - Water evaporates → cools skin
  - If sweating blocked (Ach drugs) → no sweat → vasodilation

Parasympathetic System
Major Actions

- Eyes: constricts pupils
- Lungs: constricts bronchioles
- Heart: ↓ heart rate
- GI: ↑peristalsis
- Promotes urination
  - Constricts bladder
  - Relaxes urethra
- Promotes defecation
- ✗ SLUDD
  - Salivation, lacrimation, urination, digestion, and defecation

Vascular Smooth Muscle

- Sympathetic constricts (mostly)
  - Exception is muscle, liver (vasodilates)
  - Overall effect in ↑BP
- Parasympathetic dilates
  - Indirect → endothelium releases NO
  - Lowers BP

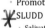

[handwritten note: Blood to muscle & liver (glyc glu)]

Anatomy

- Sympathetic ganglia
  - Paravertebral
  - T1-L5
- Parasympathetic
  - Brainstem, sacrum
  - Ganglia near target organs

Signal Transmission

- Two synapses for both systems
- First synapse (neuron 1 - neuron 2)
- Second synapse (neuron 2 - target)
- Need to know:
  - Neurotransmitters
  - Receptor types

Signal Transmission

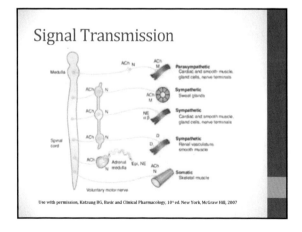

Use with permission, Katzung BG, Basic and Clinical Pharmacology, 10th ed. New York, McGraw Hill, 2007

Key Points

- NE: Main NT for sympathetic system
  - Responsible for most effects
  - Exceptions:
    - Sweat glands (ACh M)
    - Adrenal gland (ACh N)
    - Dopamine
- ACh M: Main system for parasympathetic
- ACh N: Main system for somatic muscle

Acetylcholine Synapses

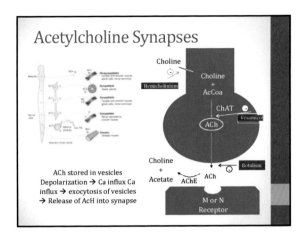

ACh stored in vesicles
Depolarization → Ca influx Ca
influx → exocytosis of vesicles
→ Release of AcH into synapse

Botulism

Blocks ACh release

- Paralytic neurotoxin → clostridium botulinum
- Three types: food, wound, infant
- Food (toxin ingestion)
  - Undercooked food
  - Canned food: anaerobic environment promotes growth
  - Watch for multiple sick adults after a meal
- Wound (bacterial growth)
  - Infection with c. botulinum
- Infant (spores)
  - Ingestion of spores → growth in infant intestine
  - Watch for contaminated honey!

Botulism

- Symptoms: 12-48 hours after ingestion
- Symptoms: 3 D's
  - Diplopia, dysphagia, dysphonia
  - Nicotinic blockade signs dominate
- Treatment:
  - Antitoxin blocks circulating toxin
  - Cannot block toxin already in nerves
  - Supportive care → toxin washout

BoTox

- Cosmetic
  - Prevents/limits wrinkles
  - Paralysis of facial muscles
- Spasms, dystonias

Adrenergic Synapses

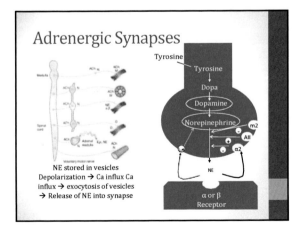

NE stored in vesicles
Depolarization → Ca influx Ca
influx → exocytosis of vesicles
→ Release of NE into synapse

Adrenergic Synapses

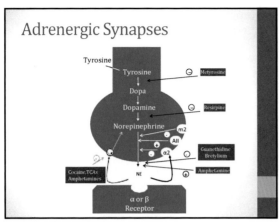

NE feedback

Cocaine Intoxication

- Inhibition of reuptake NE, dopa, serotonin
- Agitation
- Hypertension
- Dilated pupils
- Chest pain (coronary vasoconstriction)
- Look for abnormal nasal mucosa/septum

blocks sodium channels
local anesthesia

Adrenergic Receptors Subtypes

- α1 receptors in periphery
  - Peripheral vessels: Vasoconstrict (↑BP)
  - Eye: Mydriasis (dilation of pupil)
- α2 receptors in CNS
  - Presynaptic receptor
  - Feedback to nerve when NE released
  - Activation leads to ↓NE release
  - Also pancreas: inhibit insulin release

via negative feedback

Adrenergic Receptors Subtypes

- β1 receptors in heart, kidneys
  - Heart: ↑ heart rate and contractility
  - Kidneys: Stimulate renin release - JG apparatus
- β2 receptors in periphery
  - Lungs: Bronchodilate
  - Liver, muscle: vasodilation (↓BP)
  - GI: ↓motility
  - Bladder: Relaxation

Adrenergic Hemodynamics

- α1: Vasoconstriction
- α2: Vasodilation
- β1: Heart Rate
- β2: Vasodilation
- Stimulation of all receptors → ↑HR, ↑BP

Ligand-Gated Ion Channel
Nicotinic Receptors

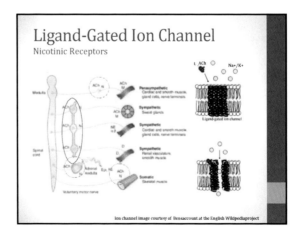

Ion channel image courtesy of Bensaccount at the English Wikipediaproject

G-Protein Linked Receptors
Muscarinic, Adrenergic Receptors

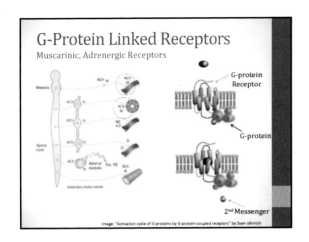

2nd Messenger

Image: "Activation cycle of G-proteins by G-protein-coupled receptors" by Sven Jähnich

G Proteins Subtypes

- Gi → inhibitory to adenylate cyclase
- Gs → stimulatory to adenylate cyclase
- Gq

Gs and Gi Systems

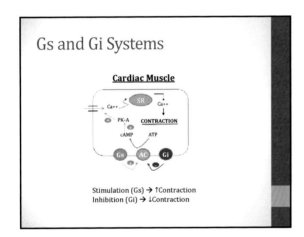

Stimulation (Gs) → ↑Contraction
Inhibition (Gi) → ↓Contraction

Gs and Gi Systems

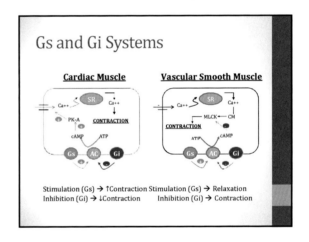

Stimulation (Gs) → ↑Contraction   Stimulation (Gs) → Relaxation
Inhibition (Gi) → ↓Contraction   Inhibition (Gi) → Contraction

Gq Systems
Cardiovascular Effects

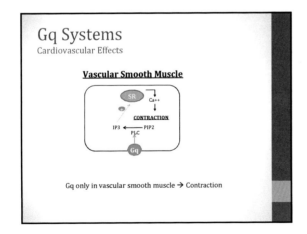

Gq only in vascular smooth muscle → Contraction

G-Protein Receptors and Types

Receptor	G protein Class
α1	q
α2	i
β1	s
β2	s
M1	q
M2	i
M3	q
D1	s
D2	i
H1	q
H2	s
V1	q
V2	s

G-Protein Subclasses

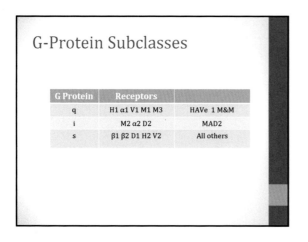

G Protein	Receptors	
q	H1 α1 V1 M1 M3	HAVe 1 M&M
i	M2 α2 D2	MAD2
s	β1 β2 D1 H2 V2	All others

Take Home Points

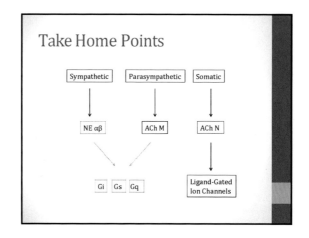

Sympathetic Parasympathetic Somatic

NE αβ ACh M ACh N

Gi Gs Gq

Ligand-Gated Ion Channels

Autonomic Drugs: Norepinephrine

Jason Ryan, MD, MPH

Adrenergic Drugs

- Amplify sympathetic system
  - Sympathomimetic drugs
  - Direct: NE receptor agonists
  - Indirect: Block NE reuptake
- Block sympathetic system
  - Adrenergic antagonists/blockers
  - Alpha blockers
  - Beta blockers

Adrenergic Activation
Hemodynamic Effects

- α1: Vasoconstriction
- α2: Vasodilation
- β1: ↑ Heart Rate/Contractility
- β2: Vasodilation

Direct Agonists

Drug	α	β1	β2	Comments
Epinephrine	+++++	++++	+++	All receptor types
Dopamine*	+++	++++	++	All receptor types
Isoproterenol		+++++	+++++	β1=β2; ↑HR ↓BP
Dobutamine	+	+++++	+++	Mostly β1; ↑HR ↓BP
Norepinephrine	+++++	+++	++	Vasoconstrictor
Phenylephrine	+++++			Vasoconstrictor

*Only Dopamine activates D1 receptors → ↑renal blood flow

Dopamine

- Does not cross blood brain barrier (no CNS effects)
- Peripheral effects highly dependent on dose
- Low dose: dopamine agonist
  - Vasodilation in kidneys
- Medium dose: beta-1 agonist
  - Increased heart rate and contractility
- High dose: alpha agonist
  - Vasoconstriction

Epinephrine

- Also dose dependent effects
- Low dose: beta-1 and beta-2 agonist
  - Increased heart rate/contractility
  - Vasodilation
- High dose: alpha agonist
  - Vasoconstriction

Other Direct Agonists

Drug	α1	α2	β1	β2	Comments
Pseudoephedrine	++	++			Nasal decongestant
Albuterol			++	++++	Asthma
Salmeterol			++	++++	COPD
Terbutaline			++	++++	OB Drug: ↓ Contractions
Ritodrine				++++	OB Drug: ↓ Contractions

Alpha Agonists
Clonidine and Methyldopa

- Used in hypertension
- Agonists to CNS α2 receptors

Alpha Agonists
Apraclonidine

- Used in glaucoma
- Agonists to α2 receptors (weak α1 activity)
- Lowers intraocular pressure

Indirect Agonists

Drug	Effect	Uses
Amphetamine	NE: Blocks reuptake, promotes release	Stimulant: Narcolepsy, obesity, ADHD
Ephedrine	NE: Promotes release	Nasal decongestant, urinary incontinence
Cocaine	NE: Blocks reuptake	Vasoconstrictor, local anesthetic

Indirect Agonists

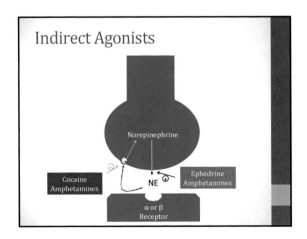

Cocaine

- Enhances **monoamine neurotransmitter activity**
  - Dopamine, Norepinephrine, Serotonin
- Blockade of presynaptic reuptake pumps
- Generalized sympathetic activation
- Also blocks Na channels in nerves (local anesthetic)

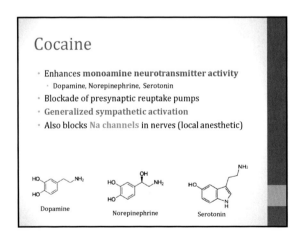

Cocaine Intoxication

- Massive alpha and beta stimulation
- Hypertension
- Tachycardia
- Classic case:
  - College student
  - Agitated, tremulous
  - Tachycardic/hypertensive
  - Chest pain (coronary spasm; increased O2 demand)

Cocaine Intoxication

- Treatment: Benzodiazepines
  - Sedatives/anxiolytics
  - Activate GABA receptors
  - Inhibitory to central nervous system
- Avoid beta blockers for chest pain/hypertension
- β2 activation blunting alpha activation
- Beta blocker → unopposed α → severe HTN

Clinical Scenarios

Case	Drug
5-year-old boy Bee sting Hives, wheezing	Anaphylaxis: Epinephrine
75-year-old man Pneumonia, hypotension	Septic shock: Norepinephrine, Phenylephrine
66-year-old man Massive myocardial infarction Hypotension	Cardiogenic Shock: Dobutamine
10-year-old boy History of asthma Wheezing, dyspnea	Asthma flare: Albuterol
22-year-old man, runny nose	Rhinitis: Pseudoephedrine, phenylephrine

Alpha Blockers
Nonselective (α1α2)

- Phenoxybenzamine (irreversible)
  - Used in pheochromocytoma
- Phentolamine (reversible)
  - Used to reverse "cheese effect"
  - MAOi drugs block breakdown neurotransmitters (depression)
  - Also block breakdown tyramine
  - Eat cheese (tyramine) → dangerous HTN
- Side Effects: hypotension, reflex tachycardia

Tyramine

Dopamine

Alpha Blockers
α1 Blockers

- Prazosin, terazosin, doxazosin, tamsulosin
- Used in hypertension, urinary retention BPH

Alpha Blockers
α2 Blockers

- Mirtazapine
- Depression drug
- Affects serotonin and NE levels in CNS

Beta Blockers

- β1-selective antagonists
  - Esmolol, Atenolol, Metoprolol
- β1β2 (nonselective)antagonists
  - Propranolol, Timolol, Nadolol
- β1β2α1
  - Carvedilol, Labetalol
- Partial-agonists
  - Pindolol, Acebutolol

Drug Experiments

- Unknown drug given
- Heart rate and blood pressure response shown
- Question: Which receptors effected by drug?

Drug Experiments
Heart Rate Effects

- β1 → tachycardia
- β2 → vasodilation → tachycardia (reflex)
- α1 → vasoconstriction → bradycardia (reflex)
- α2 → ↓ norepinephrine → bradycardia

Drug Experiments
Blood Pressure Effects

- Systolic blood pressure
  - Primary determinant: cardiac output
- Diastolic blood pressure
  - Primary determinant: peripheral resistance

Drug Experiments
Blood Pressure Effects

- Beta-1 effects
  - Increased heart rate/contractility
  - Increased cardiac output
- Main effect: **systolic** pressure goes up
  - Mean blood pressure rises

Drug Experiments
Blood Pressure Effects

- Beta-2 effects
  - Vasodilation
  - Main effect: **Diastolic** blood pressure falls
- Overall result: Mean blood pressure will fall
- Reflex tachycardia

β2   HR   MAP   DBP

Drug Experiments
Blood Pressure Effects

- Alpha-1 effects
  - Vasoconstriction
  - Main effect: **Diastolic** blood pressure rises
- Overall result: Mean blood pressure will increase
- Reflex bradycardia

$\alpha1$ HR
MAP
DBP

Drug Experiments
Blood Pressure Effects

- Alpha-2 effects
  - Blunts sympathetic nervous system
- Heart rate and MAP will fall
- Clonidine/Methyldopa used in hypertension

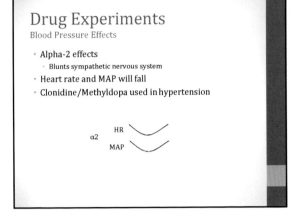

Drug Experiments

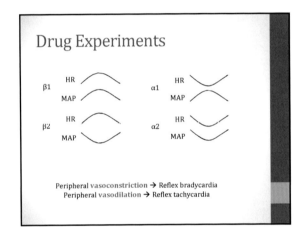

Peripheral **vasoconstriction** → Reflex bradycardia
Peripheral **vasodilation** → Reflex tachycardia

Dobutamine

- Mostly $\beta1$
- ↑ cardiac output
- ↑ heart rate
- MAP pressure usually falls
  - ↓ TPR ($\beta2$)
  - Limited $\alpha1$ effects
  - ↑ cardiac output
- Myocyte effect > SA node
- More inotropy than chronotropy

CO ↑
HR ↑
MAP ↓

Dopamine/Epinephrine

- $\beta1\beta2\alpha1$
- Effects vary with dose
- ↑ cardiac output → ↑ SBP
- ↑ heart rate
- ↑ DBP ($\alpha1$ – dose dependent)
- ↑ MAP

CO ↑
HR ↑
MAP ↑

Norepinephrine

CO ↑
HR ↑↓
MAP ↑↑

- $\alpha1\beta1$
- $\alpha1 >> \beta1$
- Major effect: **Increased TPR**
  - Increased DBP and MAP
- Heart rate effects variable
  - Some ↑ HR from $\beta1$
  - Some ↓ HR from **reflex bradycardia**
  - Can see no change in heart rate
- Cardiac output usually goes up from $\beta1$
  - Rise in SBP

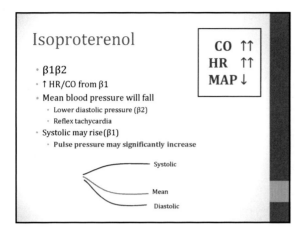

Isoproterenol

CO ↑↑
HR ↑↑
MAP ↓

- β1β2
- ↑ HR/CO from β1
- Mean blood pressure will fall
  - Lower diastolic pressure (β2)
  - Reflex tachycardia
- Systolic may rise (β1)
  - Pulse pressure may significantly increase

Systolic
Mean
Diastolic

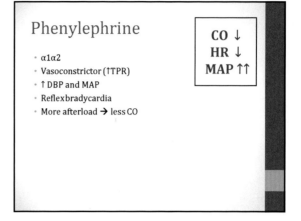

Phenylephrine

CO ↓
HR ↓
MAP ↑↑

- α1α2
- Vasoconstrictor (↑TPR)
- ↑ DBP and MAP
- Reflex bradycardia
- More afterload → less CO

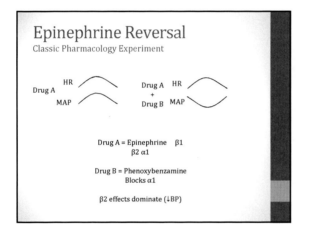

Epinephrine Reversal
Classic Pharmacology Experiment

Drug A   HR
          MAP

Drug A
+
Drug B   HR
          MAP

Drug A = Epinephrine   β1
                        β2 α1

Drug B = Phenoxybenzamine
         Blocks α1

β2 effects dominate (↓BP)

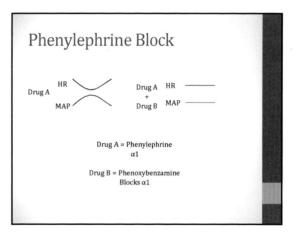

Phenylephrine Block

Drug A   HR
          MAP

Drug A
+
Drug B   HR
          MAP

Drug A = Phenylephrine
         α1

Drug B = Phenoxybenzamine
         Blocks α1

Autonomic Drugs: Acetylcholine

Jason Ryan, MD, MPH

Autonomic System

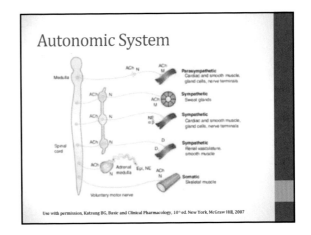

Use with permission, Katzung BG, Basic and Clinical Pharmacology, 10ᵗʰ ed. New York, McGraw Hill, 2007

Vocabulary

- Adrenergic
  - Related to norepinephrine or epinephrine
- Cholinergic
  - Related to acetylcholine
- Anti-adrenergic or anti-cholinergic

Receptors Clinical Effects

- Muscarinic
  - Parasympathetic PLUS sweat
  - No sweat = ↑temp
  - ↑temp = skin flushing
- Nicotinic
  - Blockers: paralytics

Muscarinic Agonist Effects

- Visceral smooth muscle
  - Increase GI motility
  - Nausea, vomiting, cramps, diarrhea
- Secretory glands
  - Sweating, salivation, lacrimation
- Bladder
  - Detrusor (smooth muscle) contraction: Urination

Muscarinic Agonist Effects

- Heart
  - Decreased contractility (less Ca into cells)
  - Decreased HR (less Ca in SA/AV nodes)
- Lungs
  - Bronchoconstriction
  - Wheezing, dyspnea, flare of asthma/COPD

Muscarinic Agonist Effects

- Endothelial cells
  - No direct effect on vascular smooth muscle
  - Indirectly stimulate NO release
  - Activates guanylate cyclase → less Ca → vasodilation
  - ↓BP

Acetylcholine Agonists

Drug	Actions	Uses
Bethanechol	Activates bowel and bladder	Ileus, urinary retention
Carbachol	Lowers intraocular pressure	Glaucoma, pupillary constriction
Pilocarpine	Lowers intraocular pressure	Glaucoma
Methacholine	Bronchoconstriction	Test for asthma

Acetylcholine Esterase Inhibitors

Drug	Uses
Neostigmine	Ileus, urinary retention, myasthenia gravis
Pyridostigmine	Myasthenia gravis
Edrophonium	Myasthenia gravis
Physostigmine	Anticholinergic toxicity
Donepezil	Alzheimer's

Myasthenia Gravis

- Autoimmune disease
- Antibodies block ACh receptors
- Nicotinic receptors in muscles clinically affected

Myasthenia Gravis

- Classic signs/symptoms:
  - Eye problems
  - Chewing, talking, swallowing problems
- Classic finding is fatigability
  - Repetitive movements ↓ACh levels, problem worsens
- Treatment
  - Neostigmine, Pyridostigmine, Edrophonium
  - Immunosuppressants

Myasthenia Gravis

- Exacerbations can occur for two reasons
- #1: Insufficient dose AChE inhibitor
- #2: Cholinergic crisis
  - Too much medication
  - Muscle refractory to ACh
- Tensilon test: Give edrophonium
- If muscle function improves: ↑dose
- Muscle function fails to improve: ↓dose

Lambert-Eaton Syndrome

- Similar to MG
- Paraneoplastic syndrome (small cell lung cancer)
- Antibodies against pre-synaptic Ca channels
  - Prevent ACh release
- Edrophonium test: No improvement

COPD and Peptic Ulcers

- Any cholinergic medication can worsen
- ACh agonists and AChE inhibitors
- Bronchoconstriction → COPD flare
- ↑gastric acid → ulcers

Organophosphate Poisoning

- A 44-year-old farmer presents to the ER with difficulty breathing. There is audible wheezing. He also reports diarrhea and unintentional loss of urine. He appears agitated. On exam, he has pinpoint pupils. He is sweaty, drooling, and his eyes are watery. His pulse is 30.

Organophosphate Poisoning

- Exposure to insecticides often through skin
- Irreversible block of AChE
- All acetylcholine synapses in overdrive

Organophosphate Poisoning

- ↑Muscarinic activity
  - Diarrhea, urination, bronchospasm, bradycardia, salivation (drool), lacrimation (tears)
- ↑Nicotinic activity
  - Fasciculation
- ↑CNS activity
  - Confusion, lethargy, seizures

Organophosphate Poisoning

- Treatment:
  - Atropine – Muscarinic antagonist
  - Pralidoxime – regenerates AChE
- Farmer with confusion, sweating, pinpoint pupils

ACh Antagonist Effects

- Dry skin
  - Blockade of sympathetic sweat glands
- Hyperthermia
  - Loss of sweating
- Flushing
  - Reflex vasodilation in response to hyperthermia

ACh Antagonist Effects

- Dry mouth and eyes
  - No lacrimation, salivation
- Dilated eyes
  - Can trigger acute angle closure glaucoma
- Delirium
  - Blockade of central ACh
- Red as a beet, dry as a bone, blind as a bat, mad as a hatter, and hot as a hare

Acetylcholine Antagonists
Muscarinic Blockers

Drug	Uses
Homatropine, tropicamide	Eye drugs: Dilate pupil (mydriasis)
Benztropine, Trihexyphenidyl	Parkinson's
Scopolamine	Motion Sickness
ipratropium, tiotropium	Inhalers: COPD
Oxybutynin	Urinary incontinence: Reduces bladder spasms
Glycopyrrolate	Pre-op: Reduce airway secretions

Motion Sickness

- Overstimulation of M1 and H1 → nausea/vomiting
- Scopolamine patch → blocks M1
- Also antihistamines
  - Meclizine
  - Dimenhydrinate
- Side effects: dry mouth, urinary retention, constipation

Atropine

- A 50-year-old man feels dizzy after a central line is placed in his left jugular vein. His EKG is shown below.

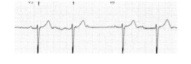

Atropine

- His is given Atropine and his dizziness resolves. His EKG converts the tracing below.

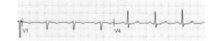

- Later that night he has pelvic discomfort and is unable to urinate.

Atropine

- Muscarinic antagonist
- Used for bradycardia and pupil dilation
- ACLS algorithm for cardiac arrest

Atropine

- Toxicity:
  - ↑temperature (no sweating)
  - Dry skin
  - Dry mouth
  - Constipation
  - Urinary retention
  - Confusion (elderly)
- Treatment: Physostigmine

Atropine

- Contraindicated in glaucoma
  - Decreases outflow of fluid
  - Sudden eye pain, halos

Gardener's Mydriasis

- Jimson weed toxin
- Anticholinergic properties (like atropine)
- Dilated pupils
- Tachycardia
- Hypertension
- Dry mouth
- Treatment: Physostigmine

ACh Synapse Poisoning

- Botulism
  - Nicotinic and muscarinic blockade
  - Paralysis dominates picture (cranial nerves/descending)
  - GI symptoms if food borne contamination
- Atropine overdose
  - Muscarinic blockade
  - No muscle effects
- Organophosphates
  - Nicotinic and muscarinic activation
  - Weakness from depolarizing blockade: fasciculations
  - Muscarinic stim: miosis, bradycardia, tears, sweat

Anticholinergic Side Effects

- Caused by many drugs
  - Tricyclic antidepressants
  - First gen antihistamines - chlorpheniramine, diphenhydramine
  - Antipsychotics
  - Anti-parkinsons
- Pupil dilation
- Dry mouth
- Constipation
- Urinary retention
- Sedation

Urinary Retention

- Common side effect anti-cholinergic drugs
- More common older men with BPH
- Watch for this after atropine, others
- Other drugs with anti-cholinergic properties
  - TCAs, Haldol

Nicotinic Blockers

- Used for paralysis in anesthesia

The Pupil

Jason Ryan, MD, MPH

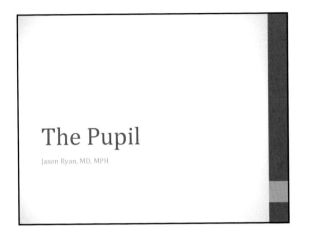

The Pupil

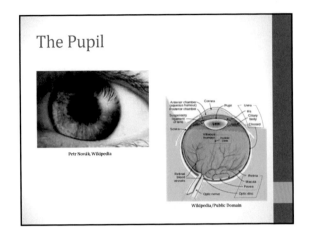

Petr Novák, Wikipedia

Wikipedia/Public Domain

Pupil

- Controls amount of light entering eye
- **Contraction = miosis**
- Dilation = mydriasis
- Under autonomic control

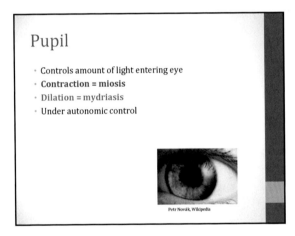

Petr Novák, Wikipedia

Iris

- Contractile structure
- Mainly smooth muscle
- Controls size of pupil
- Two muscle groups
- Circular group: **sphincter pupillae**
- Radial group: **dilator pupillae**

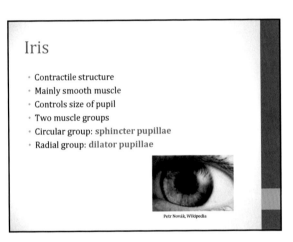

Petr Novák, Wikipedia

Iris

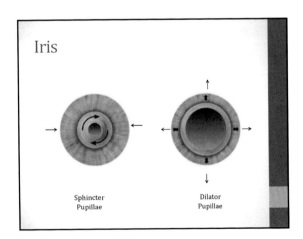

Sphincter Pupillae

Dilator Pupillae

Miosis
Pupillary contraction

- **Parasympathetic control**
- Two neuron pathway
- Begins at the **Edinger-Westphal nucleus**
  - Midbrain: Near oculomotor (CNIII) nucleus
- Nerve fibers enter orbit with cranial nerve III
- Synapse at ciliary ganglion (behind the eye)
- Ciliary ganglion signals sphincter pupillae
  - Via the short ciliary nerves
- **Muscarinic receptors (ACh)**

Miosis
Pupillary contraction

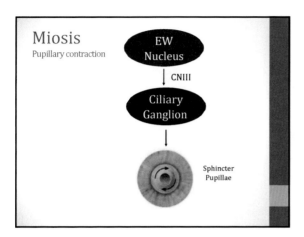

Rule of the Pupil

- Cranial nerve III lesion: eye down and out
- **Pupil dilation: Parasympathetic nerves impacted**
  - Parasympathetic fibers run on outside of nerve
  - Easily compressed by mass (Pcomm aneurysm)
- **Absence of pupillary dilation suggests ischemia**
  - CNIII ischemic nerve damage common in diabetes
  - Spares superficial fibers to pupil

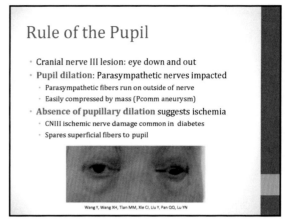

Wang Y, Wang XH, Tian MM, Xie CJ, Liu Y, Pan QQ, Lu YN

Adie's Tonic Pupil

- **Dilated pupil**
- Blocked parasympathetic innervation
- Most cases idiopathic
- Can be caused by orbit disorders of ciliary ganglion
- Tumor, inflammation, trauma, surgery, infection

Mydriasis
Pupillary dilation

- **Sympathetic control**
- Activation of dilator pupillae
  - Also inhibition of sphincter pupillae
- **Norepinephrine receptors (α1)**
- Long, three neuron chain
- Brain to spinal cord back up to eye

Mydriasis
Pupillary dilation

- #1: Post hypothalamus to spinal cord
  - Ends at ciliospinal centre of Budge (C8-T2)
- #2: Spinal cord to superior cervical ganglion
  - Exit at T1
  - Crosses apical pleura of the lung
  - Travels with cervical sympathetic chain (near subclavian)
- #3: Superior cervical ganglion to dilator pupillae
  - Courses with internal carotid artery
  - Passes through cavernous sinus

Mydriasis
Pupillary dilation

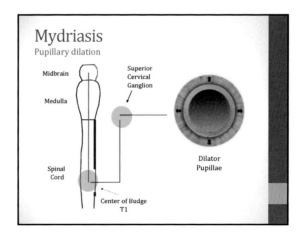

Horner Syndrome

- Disruption of sympathetic chain to face
- Small pupil (miosis)
  - Loss of sympathetic innervation → pupillary contraction
- Eyelid droop (ptosis)
  - Sympathetic system supplies superior tarsal muscle
  - Assists levator palpebrae in raising eyelid
- No sweat (anhidrosis)

Horner Syndrome
Causes

- Apical lung tumor
- Aortic dissection
- Carotid dissection
- PICA stroke (lateral medullary syndrome)

Cocaine
Diagnostic Test for Horner Syndrome

- Blocks reuptake of norepinephrine
- No effect with impaired sympathetic innervation
- Testing: Cocaine applied to eye
- Normal eye: Dilation
- Horner syndrome eye: No dilation

Anisocoria

- Difference in pupil sizes
- Seen in Horner syndrome
- CNIII palsy with pupillary involvement
- Adie's pupil

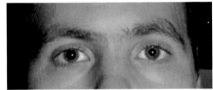

Radomil talk/Wikipedia

Pupillary Reflexes

1. Light
2. Accommodation

Pupillary Light Reflex

- Shine light in one eye → both eyes constrict
  - Illuminated eye: **direct** response
  - Opposite eye: **consensual** response
- Light signals to **pretectal nucleus (midbrain)**
- Pretectal nucleus to **bilateral EW nucleus**
- Does not involve cortex - purely a reflex of nerves

Pupillary Light Reflex

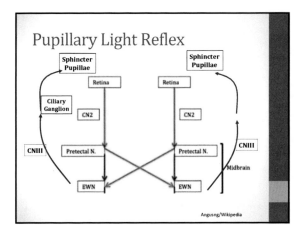

Angusng/Wikipedia

Marcus Gunn Pupil

- Relative afferent pupillary defect (RAPD)
- Light shone in 1 eye produces less constriction
- Diagnosed by the "Swinging Flashlight Test"

Swinging Flashlight Test

- Shine light in one eye
- Should see bilateral constriction
- Swing light to other eye
- Constriction should remain same
- If constriction less (dilation) → APD

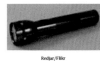

Redjar/Flikr

Marcus Gunn Pupil

- Caused by lesion in "afferent" light reflex limb
  - Problem sensing light appropriately
- Many potential causes: retina, optic nerve
- Classic cause: **Optic neuritis**
  - Inflammatory, demyelinating disorder
  - Commonly occurs in **multiple sclerosis**

Accommodation

- Changes optical power to focus on near objects
- Ciliary muscle changes shape of lens
- Associated with miosis (pupillary constriction)

Accommodation Reflex

- #1 Convergence:
  - Eyes move medially to track object
- #2 Accommodation
  - Shape of lens changes
  - Focal point maintained on retina
- #3 Miosis
  - Pupil constricts
  - Block entry of divergent light rays from near object
- Complex reflex circuit: involves visual cortex

Argyll Robertson Pupil

- "Prostitute's pupil"
- Strongly associated with neurosyphilis (tertiary)
- Bilateral, small pupils
- **No constriction to light**
- **Constriction to accommodation**
- "Light-near dissociation"
- Believed to involve pretectal nucleus
  - Part of light reflex; not part of accommodation reflex

PERRLA

- Documentation of normal pupil exam
- Pupils equal, round, reactive to light and accommodation

The Lens

Jason Ryan, MD, MPH

The Lens

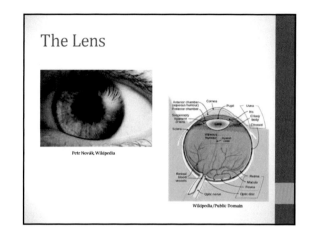

Petr Novák, Wikipedia

Wikipedia/Public Domain

How Lenses Work
Refraction

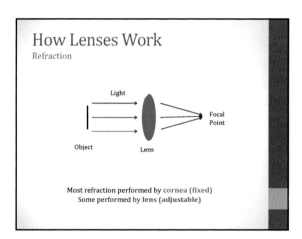

Most refraction performed by cornea (fixed)
Some performed by lens (adjustable)

The Lens

- Surrounded by a capsule with **type IV collagen**
- Avascular
  - Nutrients via diffusion
- Contains elongated fiber cells
- **Anaerobic metabolism**
  - Principle source of energy production
  - Glucose → lactic acid

Accommodation

- Lens modifies shape to focus on near objects
- Lens changes optical power of eye

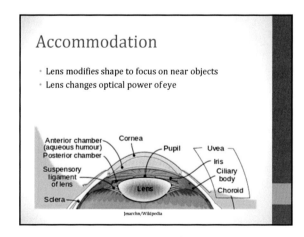

Accommodation

- Ciliary muscle: Smooth muscle within ciliary body
- Changes shape of lens
- Circular muscle – surrounds lens
- Connected to lens by ligaments (zonules)

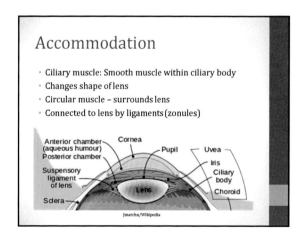

Accommodation

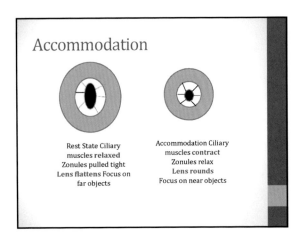

Rest State Ciliary muscles relaxed Zonules pulled tight **Lens flattens** Focus on far objects

Accommodation Ciliary muscles contract Zonules relax **Lens rounds** Focus on near objects

Lens of the Eye

- Far objects
  - Ciliary relax
  - Lens flatter
- Near objects
  - Ciliary contract
  - Lens rounder

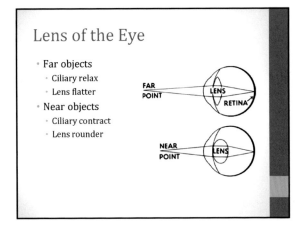

Presbyopia

- Lens stiffens with age
- Can't focus on near objects (reading)

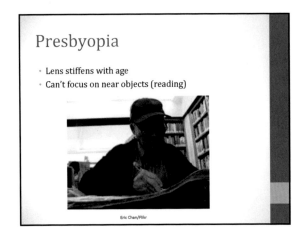

Eric Chan/Flikr

Accommodation Reflex

- 3 reflex responses as object moves closer to eye
- #1 Convergence:
  - Eyes move medially to track object
- #2 Miosis
  - Pupil constricts
  - Block entry of divergent light rays from near object
- #3 Accommodation
  - Shape of lens changes
  - Focal point maintained on retina

Refractive Errors

- Impaired vision due to abnormal focal point of eye
- Improved with glasses or contact lenses

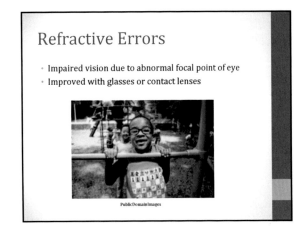

PublicDomainImages

Refractive Errors

- Corneal curvature must match eye size
- Failure to match = refractive error

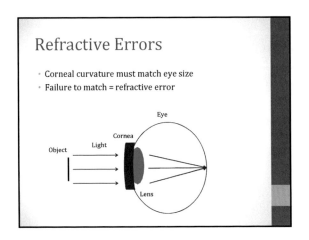

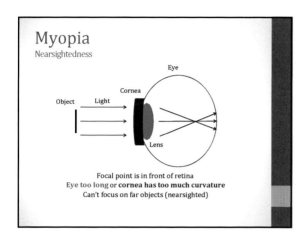

Myopia
Nearsightedness

Focal point is in front of retina
Eye too long or **cornea has too much curvature**
Can't focus on far objects (nearsighted)

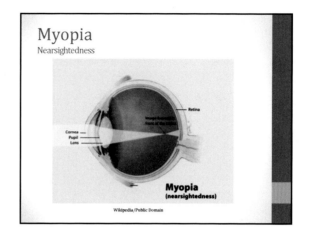

Myopia
Nearsightedness

Wikipedia/Public Domain

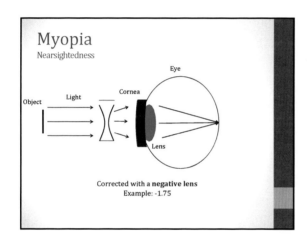

Myopia
Nearsightedness

Corrected with a **negative lens**
Example: -1.75

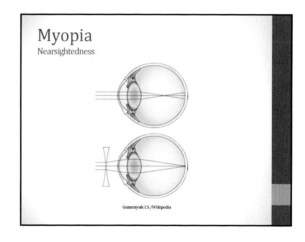

Myopia
Nearsightedness

Gumenyuk I.S./Wikipedia

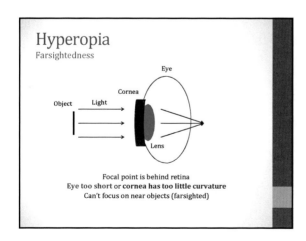

Hyperopia
Farsightedness

Focal point is behind retina
Eye too short or **cornea has too little curvature**
Can't focus on near objects (farsighted)

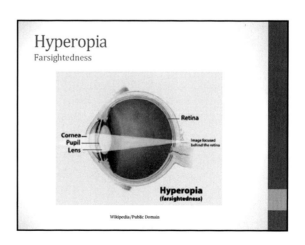

Hyperopia
Farsightedness

Wikipedia/Public Domain

Hyperopia
Farsightedness

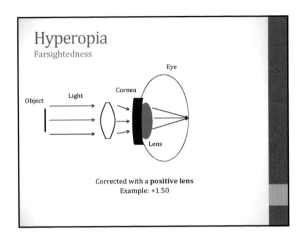

Corrected with a **positive lens**
Example: +1.50

Hyperopia
Farsightedness

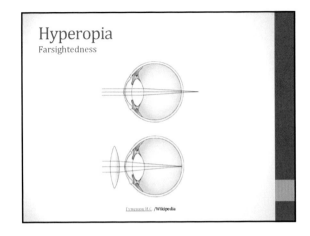

Гуменюк И.С. /Wikipedia

Astigmatism

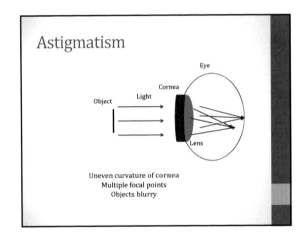

Uneven curvature of cornea
Multiple focal points
Objects blurry

Astigmatism

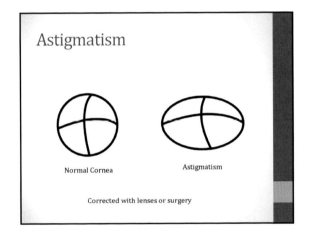

Corrected with lenses or surgery

Ectopia Lentis

- **Dislocation** of lens
- Commonly due to trauma
- Rarely associated with systemic disease
- Can occur as ocular manifestation of systemic disease

Ectopia Lentis

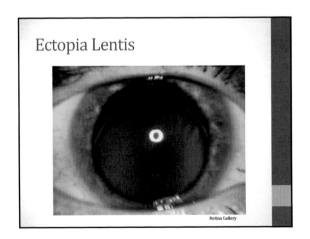

Retina Gallery

Ectopia Lentis

- **Marfan Syndrome**
  - Most commonly associated systemic condition
  - Autosomal dominant disorder; fibrillin defect
  - Tall, long wing span
  - 50-80% of cases have lens dislocation
  - Classically upward/outward lens dislocation
- Homocystinuria
  - Cystathionine β synthase deficiency
  - Markedly elevated homocysteine levels
  - Marfanoid body habitus
  - Mental retardation
  - Classically downward/inward lens dislocation

Cataracts

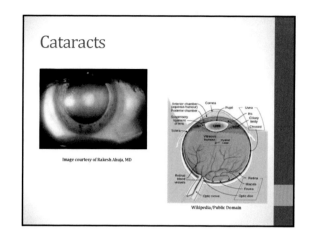

Image courtesy of Rakesh Ahuja, MD

Wikipedia/Public Domain

Cataracts

- **Opacification** of lens
- Painless
- Lead to ↓ vision
- Treated with surgery

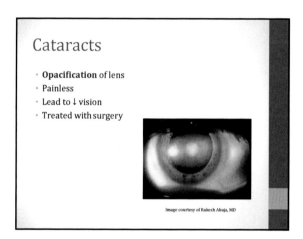

Image courtesy of Rakesh Ahuja, MD

Cataracts
Risk Factors

- Older age
- Smoking
- Alcohol
- Excessive sunlight
- Corticosteroids
- Trauma, infection

Aldose Reductase
Polyol Pathway

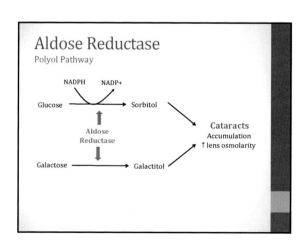

Diabetes
Cataract Risk Factor

- Glucose can be metabolized to **sorbitol** in lens

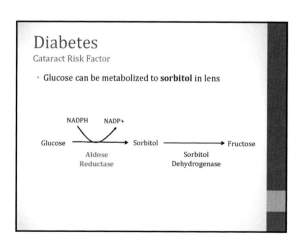

115

Galactose Disorders

- Classic Galactosemia
  - Presents in infancy
  - Live failure
  - Cataracts
- Galactokinase deficiency
  - Milder form of galactosemia
  - Main problem: cataracts as child/young adult

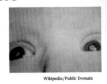

Wikipedia/Public Domain

$$\text{Galactose} \xrightarrow{\text{Aldose Reductase}} \text{Galactitol}$$

TORCH Infections

- Can lead to cataracts
- Classically part of **congenital rubella syndrome**
  - Deafness
  - Cardiac malformations
  - "Blueberry muffin" skin (extramedullary hematopoiesis)

The Retina

Jason Ryan, MD, MPH

Retina and Macula

- Retina
  - Inner layer of eye
  - Contain photosensitive cells: rods and cones
  - Major blood supply via choroid
- Macula
  - Oval-shaped area near center of retina
  - Contains fovea (largest amount of cone cells)
  - High-resolution, color vision
- Both structures essential for normal vision

Retina and Macula

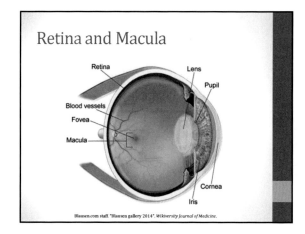

Blausen.com staff. "Blausen gallery 2014". *Wikiversity Journal of Medicine.*

Fundoscopy

- Fundus = back of eye opposite lens
- Includes retina, optic disc, macula
- "Fundoscopy" = visual examination of fundus

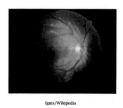

Ignis/Wikipedia

Retinitis Pigmentosa

- Inherited retinal disorder
- Visual loss usually begins in childhood
- Loss of **photoreceptors (rods and cones)**
- Night and peripheral vision lost progressively
- Constricted visual field
- No cure – most patients legal blind by age 40

Retinitis Pigmentosa
Fundoscopy

- Intraretinal pigmentation in a **bone-spicule pattern**
- Form in retina where photoreceptors are missing

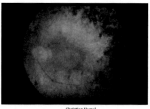

Christian Hamel

Retinitis

- Retinal edema/necrosis
- Floaters, ↓ vision
- Classic cause: **Cytomegalovirus (CMV)**
- Usually in **HIV/AIDS** (low CD4 <50)
- Also in **transplant patients** on immunosuppression

Retinitis
Fundoscopy

- Retinal hemorrhages
- Whitish appearance to retina

Wikipedia/Public Domain

Diabetic Retinopathy

- Can cause blindness among diabetics
- Pericyte degeneration
  - Cells that wrap capillaries
  - Microaneurysms
  - Rupture → hemorrhage
- Annual screening for prevention

Diabetic Retinopathy
Nonproliferative retinopathy

- Most common form of diabetic retinopathy (95%)
- "Background retinopathy"

Diabetic Retinopathy
Nonproliferative retinopathy

- Microaneurysms (earliest sign)
- "Dot-and-blot hemorrhages"
  - Damaged capillary → leakage of fluid
- Cotton-wool spots
  - Nerve infarctions
  - Occlusion of precapillary arterioles
  - Also seen in hypertension

Diabetic Retinopathy
Nonproliferative retinopathy

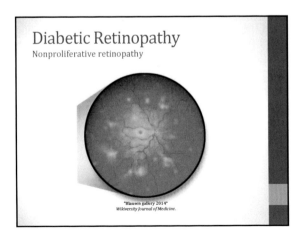

"Blausen gallery 2014"
Wikiversity Journal of Medicine.

Diabetic Retinopathy
Nonproliferative retinopathy

- Hard exudates/macular edema
  - Macular swelling
  - Yellow exudates of fatty lipids
  - Can lead to blindness in diabetics

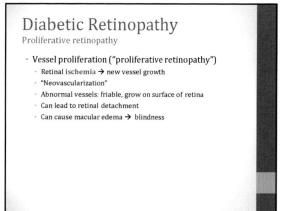

National Eye Institute, National Institutes of Health
Public Domain

Diabetic Retinopathy
Proliferative retinopathy

- Vessel proliferation ("proliferative retinopathy")
  - Retinal ischemia → new vessel growth
  - "Neovascularization"
  - Abnormal vessels: friable, grow on surface of retina
  - Can lead to retinal detachment
  - Can cause macular edema → blindness

Diabetic Retinopathy
Proliferative retinopathy

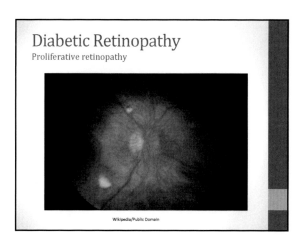

Wikipedia/Public Domain

Diabetic Retinopathy
Proliferative retinopathy

- Treatments:
  - Photocoagulation (laser → stops vessel growth)
  - Vitrectomy (bleeding/debris)
  - Anti-VEGF inhibitors (intravitreal injections; ranibizumab)

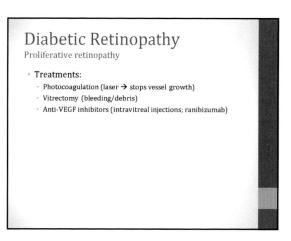

Retinal Detachment

- Retina peels away from underlying layer
- Loss of connection to choroid → ischemia
- Photoreceptors (rods/cones) degenerate
- Vision loss (curtain drawn down)
- Surgical emergency

Retinal Detachment
Fundoscopy

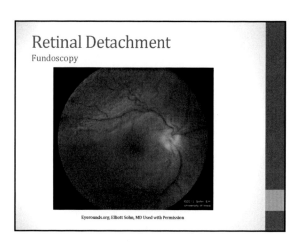

Eyerounds.org; Elliott Sohn, MD Used with Permission

Retinal Detachment

- Posterior vitreous membrane detachment
  - Often precedes retinal detachment
  - Vitreous shrinks with age → can pull on retina
  - May cause retinal holes/tears
  - Floaters (black spots)
  - Flashes of light

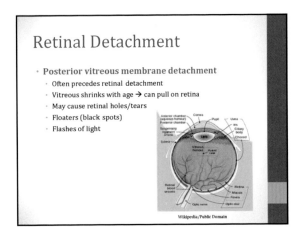

Wikipedia/Public Domain

Retinal Detachment
Risk Factors

- Myopia (near-sightedness)
  - Larger eyes; thinner retinas
- Prior eye surgery or trauma
- Proliferative diabetic retinopathy

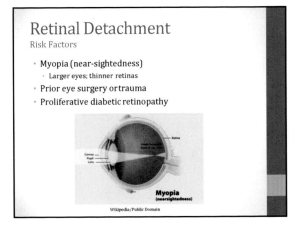

Myopia
(nearsightedness)

Wikipedia/Public Domain

Retinal Vein Occlusion

- Central or branch of retinal vein
- Can lead to visual loss

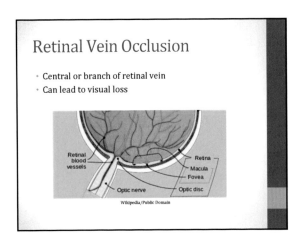

Wikipedia/Public Domain

Retinal Vein Occlusion

- Branch retinal vein occlusion (BRVO)
  - Compression of the branch vein by retinal arterioles
  - Occurs at arteriovenous crossing points
  - Associated with arteriosclerosis
  - Sclerotic arterioles compress veins in an arteriovenous sheath
- Central retinal vein occlusion (CRVO)
  - Usually a primary thrombus disorder

Retinal Vein Occlusion
Fundoscopy

- Engorged retinal veins and hemorrhages

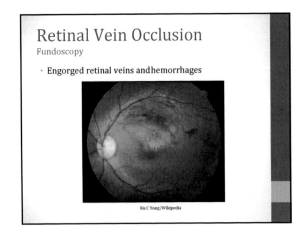

Ku C Yong/Wikipedia

Retinal Artery Occlusion

- Leads to formation of a "cherry red spot"
  - Red circular area of macula surrounded by halo
  - Also seen in Tay Sachs Disease (lysosomal storage disease)
- Commonly caused by carotid artery atherosclerosis
  - Internal carotid → ophthalmic → retinal
- Cardiac source (thrombus)
- Giant cell arteritis

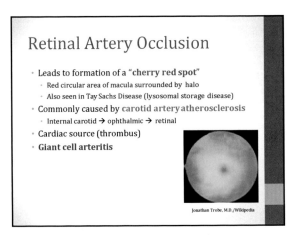

Jonathan Trobe, M.D./Wikipedia

Papilledema

- Optic disc swelling
- Due to ↑ intracranial pressure
  - i.e. mass effect
- Usually bilateral
- Blurred margins optic disc on fundoscopy

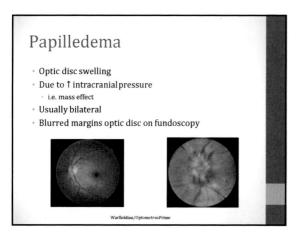

Warfieldian/OptometrusPrime

Macula

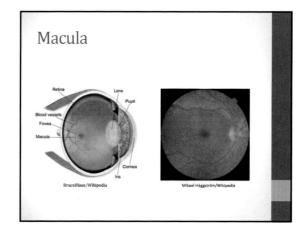

BruceBlaus/Wikipedia   Mikael Häggström/Wikipedia

Macular Degeneration

- Macula = central vision
- Degeneration → visual disruption
  - Distortion (metamorphopsia)
  - Loss of central vision (central scotomas)

Macular Degeneration

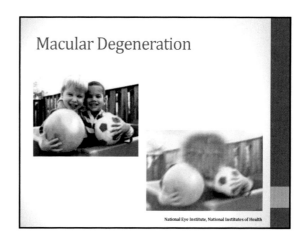

National Eye Institute, National Institutes of Health

Macular Degeneration

- Dry
  - More common (80%)
  - Slowly progressive symptoms
- Wet
  - Less common (10-15%)
  - Symptoms may develop rapidly (days/weeks)

Dry Macular Degeneration

- **Bruch's membrane**
  - Innermost layer of the choroid
  - Between choroid and retina
- **Retinal pigment epithelium**
  - Retina layer beneath photoreceptors
  - Next to choroid (Bruch's membrane)

Dry Macular Degeneration

- Accumulation of **drusen**
  - Yellow extracellular material
  - Form between Bruch's membrane and RPE
- Gradual ↓ in vision
- No specific treatment
- Vitamins and antioxidant supplements may prevent

Drusen

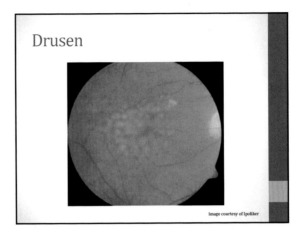

Image courtesy of Ipoliker

Wet Macular Degeneration

- Break in Bruch's membrane
- Blood vessels form beneath retina
- Leakage/hemorrhage
- Can progress rapidly to vision loss
- Treatments:
  - Laser therapy
  - Anti-VEGF (ranibizumab)

Macular Degeneration

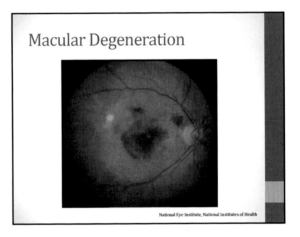

National Eye Institute, National Institutes of Health

Eye Movements

Jason Ryan, MD, MPH

Eye Movement

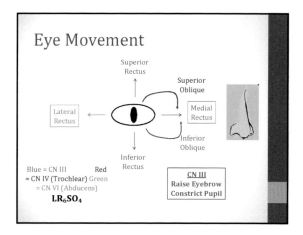

Superior
Rectus

Superior
Oblique

Lateral
Rectus

Medial
Rectus

Inferior
Oblique

Inferior
Rectus

Blue = CN III   Red
= CN IV (Trochlear) Green
= CN VI (Abducens)
LR_6SO_4

CN III
Raise Eyebrow
Constrict Pupil

Eye Nerve Palsies

- Oculomotor (III)
- Trochlear (IV)
- Abducens (VI)
- Many causes: strokes, tumors, aneurysms

Terminology

- Move eye away from nose
  - Lateral
  - Abduction
- Move eye toward nose
  - Medial
  - Adduction

Diplopia

- Two different images of same object
- Diplopia due to nerve palsies is **binocular**
  - Resolves when one eye is covered
  - Monocular diplopia: usually lens problem (astigmatism)

Jonathan Trobe, M.D./Wikipedia

Oculomotor (III)

- Moves eye up and medially
  - Up (superior rectus)
  - Medial (medial rectus)
- Elevates eyelid (levator palpebrae)
- Pupillary constriction (sphincter pupillae)
  - Parasympathetic fibers from Edinger-Westphal nucleus

Oculomotor Nerve Palsy

- Effected side
  - Eye down, out
  - Ptosis (eyelid droop)
  - Pupil dilated

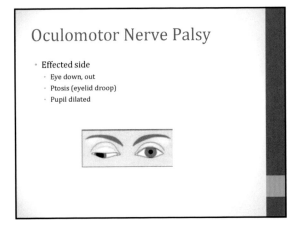

Rule of the Pupil

- Cranial nerve III lesion: eye down and out
- **Pupil dilation:** Parasympathetic nerves impacted
  - Parasympathetic fibers run on outside of nerve
  - Easily compressed by mass (Pcomm aneurysm)
- **Absence of pupillary dilation** suggests ischemia
  - CNIII ischemic nerve damage common in diabetes
  - Spares superficial fibers to pupil

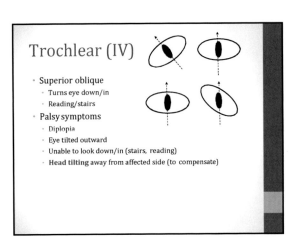

Wang Y, Wang XH, Tian MM, Xie CJ, Liu Y, Pan QQ, Lu YN

Trochlear (IV)

- Superior oblique
  - Turns eye down/in
  - Reading/stairs
- Palsy symptoms
  - Diplopia
  - Eye tilted outward
  - Unable to look down/in (stairs, reading)
  - **Head tilting** away from affected side (to compensate)

Abducens (VI)

- Lateral rectus
- Affected eye may be pulled medially at rest
- Problems worse on horizontal gaze
- Affected eye can't move laterally

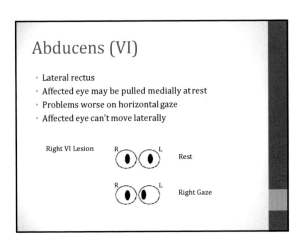

Right VI Lesion   R   L   Rest

R   L   Right Gaze

Estropia

- Type of strabismus (misalignment of the eyes)
- Inward turning of one or both eyes
- Can be seen in CN VI palsy

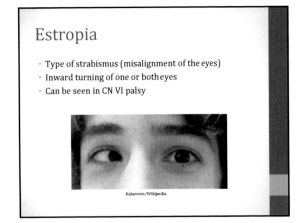

Kakawere/Wikipedia

Pseudotumor Cerebri

- High intracranial pressure (ICP) can cause CN VI palsy
- Nerve course highly susceptible to pressure forces
- Sometimes bilateral palsy
- May see papilledema on fundoscopy
- Classic patient:
  - Overweight woman
  - Childbearing age
  - Headaches

Visual Fields

Jason Ryan, MD, MPH

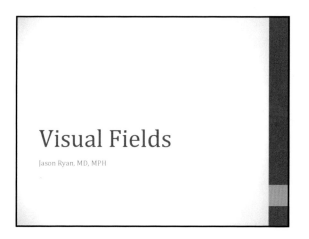

Visual Fields

- Divided into four quadrants for each eye
- Quadrants tested individually

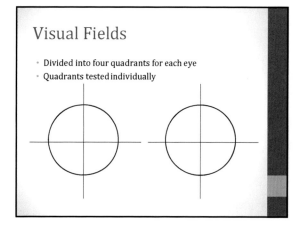

Visual System

1. Optic Nerve
2. Optic Chiasm
3. Optic Track
4. Baum's Loop
5. Meyer's Loop

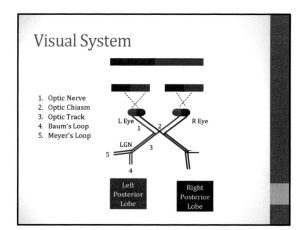

Visual System
Key Points

- Left side of world → right cortex
- Right side of world → left cortex
- Optic nerve carries signals from right/left retina
- Optic chiasm
  - Crossing of fibers from middle of both retina
  - Carrying signals from lateral (temporal) images

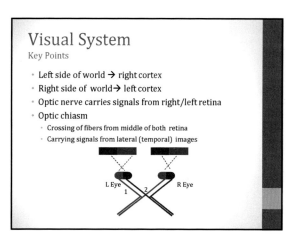

Visual System
Key Points

- Lateral geniculate nucleus
  - Found in thalamus
  - Major termination site of retinal projections
- Two projections LGN → visual cortex
  - Meyer's loop (temporal lobe)
  - Baum's loop (parietal lobe)

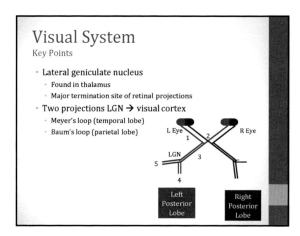

Anopia

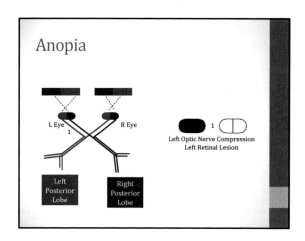

Left Optic Nerve Compression
Left Retinal Lesion

Optic Neuritis

- Inflammatory, demyelinating disease
- Acute monocular visual loss
- Highly associated with MS
  - Presenting feature 15 to 20%
  - Occurs 50% during course of illness

Amaurosis Fugax

- Painless, transient vision loss in one eye
- Classic description: **curtain shade** over vision
- Damage to optic nerve or retina
- Symptom of TIA
- Often embolism to retinal artery
- Common source is carotid artery

Bitemporal Hemianopsia

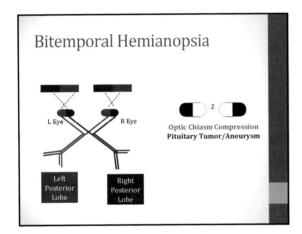

L Eye   R Eye

Optic Chiasm Compression
Pituitary Tumor/Aneurysm

Left
Posterior
Lobe

Right
Posterior
Lobe

Bitemporal Hemianopsia

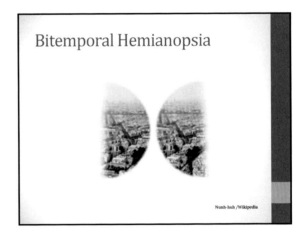

Nunh-huh /Wikipedia

Homonymous Hemianopsia

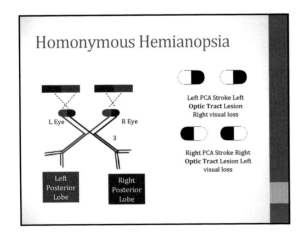

L Eye   R Eye

Left PCA Stroke Left
Optic Tract Lesion
Right visual loss

Right PCA Stroke Right
Optic Tract Lesion Left
visual loss

Left
Posterior
Lobe

Right
Posterior
Lobe

Homonymous Hemianopsia

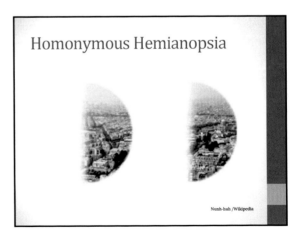

Nunh-huh /Wikipedia

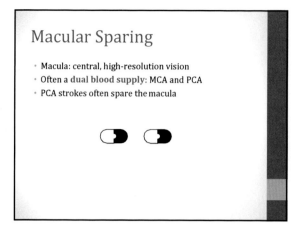

Macular Sparing

- Macula: central, high-resolution vision
- Often a **dual blood supply**: MCA and PCA
- PCA strokes often spare the macula

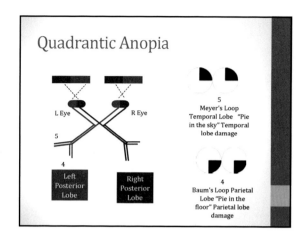

Quadrantic Anopia

L Eye   R Eye

5

4
Left Posterior Lobe   Right Posterior Lobe

5
Meyer's Loop
Temporal Lobe   "Pie in the sky" Temporal lobe damage

4
Baum's Loop Parietal Lobe "Pie in the floor" Parietal lobe damage

Gaze Palsies

Jason Ryan, MD, MPH

Conjugate Gaze

- Movement of both eyes at same time
- Looking right or left with both eyes
- Tracking objects
- Conjugate gaze palsy
  - Eyes cannot move in same direction
  - Results in diplopia

Conjugate Gaze

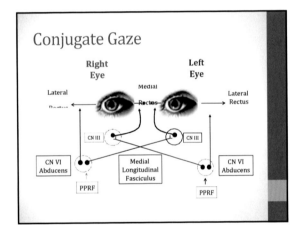

Pons

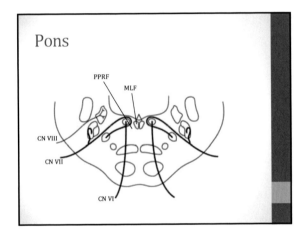

Conjugate Gaze
Summary

- Paramedian pontine reticular formation
  - Initiates lateral gaze from brainstem
  - Located in pons
- Medial longitudinal fasciculus
  - Signal transmission to opposite side
- Requires functioning CN III and CN VI

Internuclear Ophthalmoplegia

- **Horizontal** gaze disorder
- Weak adduction (medial movement) of one eye
- Affected eye cannot move toward nose
- Unaffected eye develops nystagmus
- Caused by **lesions of the MLF**
- Convergence is usually spared
  - Different neural pathway
  - CN III working normally

Internuclear Ophthalmoplegia
Example: Left INO

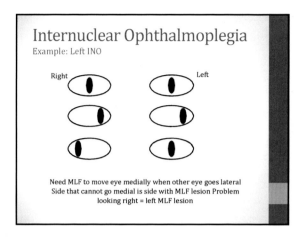

Need MLF to move eye medially when other eye goes lateral
Side that cannot go medial is side with MLF lesion Problem
looking right = left MLF lesion

Internuclear Ophthalmoplegia

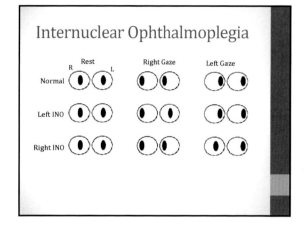

MLF Syndrome

- Lost MLF input to oculomotor nucleus on lateral gaze
- Adducting eye unable to move medially past midline
- Abducting eye: Monocular horizontal nystagmus
  - Abducting eye moves smoothly laterally
  - Followed by rapid movement back to midline (saccade)

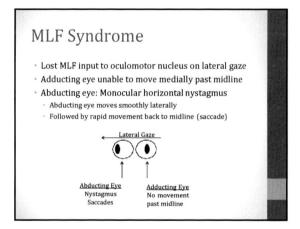

MLF Syndrome

- Commonly occurs in multiple sclerosis
- MLF is highly myelinated

Abducens (VI) Nerve Palsy

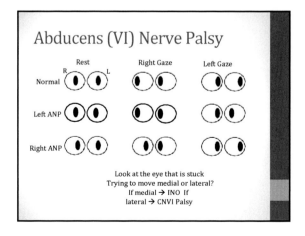

Look at the eye that is stuck
Trying to move medial or lateral?
If medial → INO If
lateral → CNVI Palsy

PPRF Lesions

- Ipsilateral Gaze Palsy
- Paralysis of conjugate gaze to side of lesion
  - Can't look to side of lesion
  - Left PPRF coordinates leftward gaze
- Preservation of convergence
- Medial pons lesions

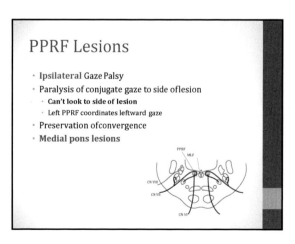

Abducens (VI) Nucleus Lesion

- Same as PPRF lesion
- Loss of lateral gaze

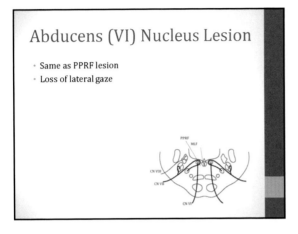

One and a Half Syndrome

- Damage to **PPRF and MLF**
- INO plus loss of lateral gaze to affected side
- Convergence spared
- Side with frozen eye has lesion

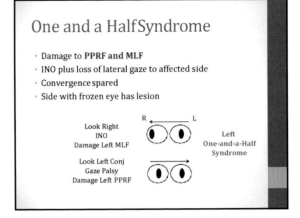

Frontal Eye Fields

- Region of **frontal cortex** (Brodmann area 8)
- Projections to contralateral PPRF

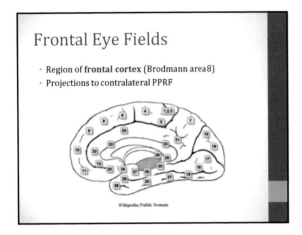

Wikipedia/Public Domain

Frontal Eye Fields

- Normal gaze central due to equal FEF activation
- **Lesion: Both eyes deviate to side of lesion**
- Stimulation: Both eyes deviate to opposite side
  - Can be seen in frontal lobe seizures

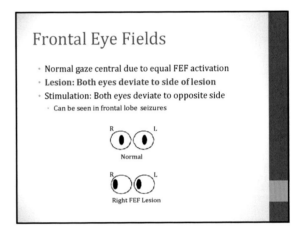

Gaze Palsy Summary

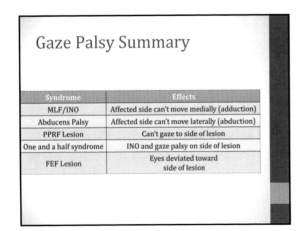

Syndrome	Effects
MLF/INO	Affected side can't move medially (adduction)
Abducens Palsy	Affected side can't move laterally (abduction)
PPRF Lesion	Can't gaze to side of lesion
One and a half syndrome	INO and gaze palsy on side of lesion
FEF Lesion	Eyes deviated toward side of lesion

Structural Eye Disorders

Jason Ryan, MD, MPH

Eye Structures

- Pupil/Iris
- Lens
- Sclera
- Conjunctiva
- Cornea
- Uvea
- Retina/Macula

Sclera and Cornea

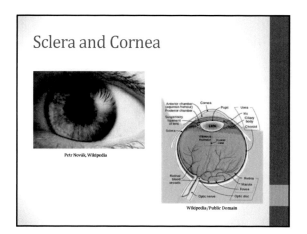

Petr Novák, Wikipedia

Wikipedia/Public Domain

Sclera and Cornea

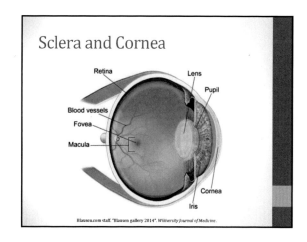

Blausen.com staff. "Blausen gallery 2014". *Wikiversity Journal of Medicine.*

Sclera

- Composed of collagen
- Rigid structure – stabilizes eyeball
- **Extraocular muscles** insertion site
- Avascular
- Nutrients from episclera and choroid

Wikipedia/Public Domain

Scleritis

- Inflammation of sclera
- Dark red eyes
- Severe "boring" pain with eye movement
- Potentially blinding

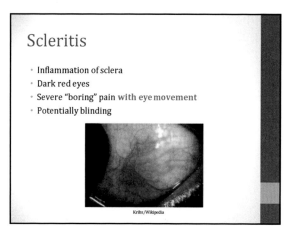

Kribz/Wikipedia

Scleritis

- 50% cases associated with systemic disease
- **Rheumatoid arthritis is most common**

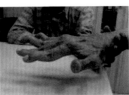

Phoenix119/Wikipedia

Episcleritis

- Acute inflammation
- Episclera layer only
- Usually idiopathic
- Tearing
- Localized redness
- Mild or no pain
- Usually self-limited
- Also associated with **rheumatoid arthritis**

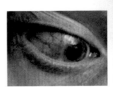

Asagan/Wikipedia

Keratitis

- Corneal inflammation
- Bacterial/viral/fungal
- **Contact lens wearers**
- Pain/Photophobia
- Red eye
- Foreign body sensation
- Sight threatening disorder

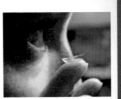

איתן טל

Corneal Abrasion

- Common among contact lens wearers
- Painful (due to superficial cornea nerve endings)
- Visualized with fluorescein dye and blue light
- Can become infected with **pseudomonas**
- Often treated with **ciprofloxacin** eye drops

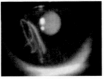

Chricres/Slideshare

HSV-1

- Causes herpes labialis
- Can also cause keratoconjunctivitis
  - Infection of cornea/conjunctiva
  - Pain, redness, discharge
- Most ocular disease is recurrent HSV
  - Reactivation after establishment of viral latency

Conjunctiva

Lady Weaxzezz/Wikipedia

Conjunctivitis

- Viral, bacterial, allergic
- Conjunctival injection
- Discharge
- Commonest "red eye"

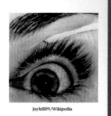

Joyhill09/Wikipedia

Conjunctivitis

- Viral causes (80%)
  - Adenovirus
  - Measles
  - HSV-1
- Bacterial causes
  - S. Aureus
  - H. influenza
  - Neisseria
  - Chlamydia

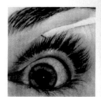

Image courtesy of Joyhill09

Adenovirus

- 65% to 90% viral conjunctivitis
- Watery discharge
- Non-enveloped, DNA virus
- Also causes pharyngitis, pneumonia

Adenovirus

- Very stable - survive on surfaces
- Transmission:
  - Aerosol droplets
  - Fecal-oral
  - Contact with contaminated surfaces

Measles Virus
Rubeola

- Paramyxovirus
- Enveloped, RNA virus
- Cough, Coryza, Conjunctivitis
- Maculopapular rash
- Koplik spots in mouth

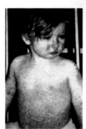

Wikipedia/Public Domain

Bacterial Conjunctivitis

- Copious purulent discharge
- Adults:
  - Staph aureus, S pneumonia, H influenzae
- Children
  - H influenzae, S pneumoniae, and Moraxella catarrhalis

Neonatal Conjunctivitis

- Ophthalmia neonatorum
- Neisseria gonorrhea or Chlamydia
- Infection from passage through birth canal
- Untreated can lead to visual impairment
- Prophylaxis: Erythromycin ophthalmic ointment

Reactive Arthritis

- Autoimmune arthritis triggered by infection
- Intestinal infections
  - Salmonella, Shigella, Campylobacter, Yersinia, C. Difficile
- Chlamydia trachomatis
- Classic triad (Reiter's syndrome)
  - Arthritis
  - Conjunctivitis (red eye, discharge)
  - Urethritis (dysuria, frequency)

Allergic Conjunctivitis

- Bilateral, itchy, watery eyes
- Type I hypersensitivity reaction
- Histamine release
- Treatment: antihistamines

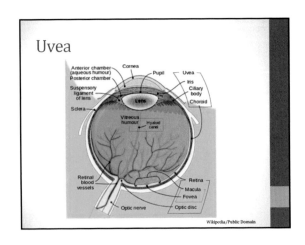

Eddie314/Wikipedia

Uvea

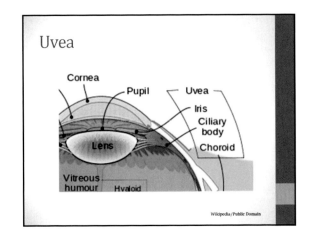

Wikipedia/Public Domain

Uvea

Wikipedia/Public Domain

Uveitis

- Uveal coat inflammation
  - Iris, ciliary body, choroid
  - White cells in uvea

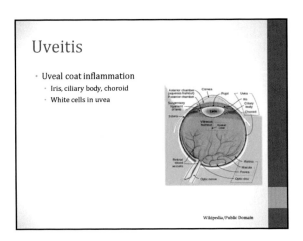

Wikipedia/Public Domain

Uveitis

Terminology

- Anterior uveitis
  - Iritis; Iridocyclitis
- Intermediate uveitis
  - Vitreous humor inflammation
- Posterior uveitis
  - Chorioretinal inflammation

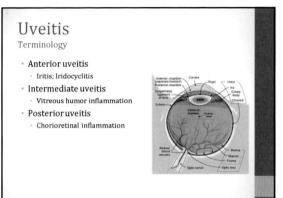

Wikipedia/Public Domain

Uveitis

Symptoms

- Anterior uveitis: pain, redness
- Posterior uveitis: painless, floaters, ↓ vision

Uveitis

Causes

- Can be infectious
  - Often agents that infect CNS
  - HSV, CMV, Toxoplasmosis, Syphilis
- Often associated with systemic inflammatory disease

Uveitis

Associations

- Ankylosing spondylitis
- Reactive arthritis
- Juvenile idiopathic arthritis
- Rheumatoid arthritis
- Sarcoid
- Psoriatic arthritis
- Inflammatory bowel disease

Hypopyon

- Inflammatory infiltrate in anterior chamber
- Seen in endophthalmitis
  - Inflammation of aqueous and/or vitreous humor
- Can be seen in keratitis, uveitis
- Bacterial or sterile

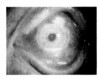

EyeMD (Rakesh Ahuja, M.D.).

Glaucoma

Jason Ryan, MD, MPH

Aqueous Humor

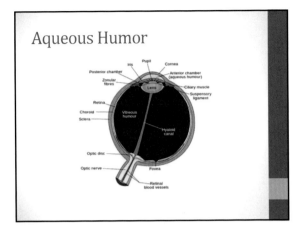

Aqueous Humor

- Ciliary muscle (accommodation) epithelium
  - Produces aqueous humor
  - Sympathetic stim (β receptors)
- Trabecular meshwork
  - Drains aqueous humor from anterior chamber
- Canal of Schlemm
  - Drains aqueous humor from trabecular meshwork

Aqueous Humor

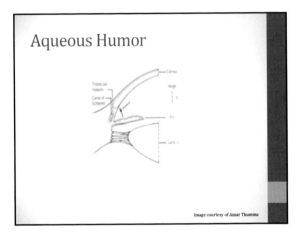

Image courtesy of Amar Thumma

Intraocular Pressure

- Measured by tonometry
- Determined by amount of aqueous humor

Intraocular Pressure

- Parasympathetic system (M)
  - Constricts ciliary muscle
  - Allows fluid to drain
  - ↓pressure
- Sympathetic (β2)
  - Produces fluid
  - Allows the eye to focus during fight/flight
  - More fluid = ↑pressure

Glaucoma

- High intraocular pressure
- Results in optic neuropathy
- Visual loss: peripheral first, then central
- Two types:
  - Open angle
  - Closed angle

The Angle

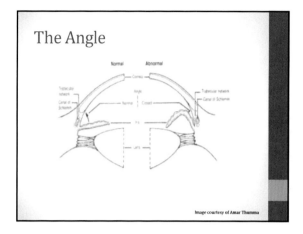

Image courtesy of Amar Thumma

Closed Angle Glaucoma

- Angle for drainage suddenly closes
- Abrupt onset
- Painful, red eye
- Blurred vision with halos
- Eye is firm ("rock hard")

"A human eye" courtesy of 8thstar and Wikipedia

Closed Angle Glaucoma

- Symptoms can be triggered when pupil dilates
  - Entering dark room
  - Drug with dilating side effect (scopolamine, atropine)
- Ophthalmologic emergency

Closed Angle Glaucoma

- Medical treatment:
  - Acetazolamide (carbonic anhydrase inhibitor)
  - Mannitol (osmotic diuretic)
  - Timolol (BB)
  - Pilocarpine (M agonist)
- Eye surgery

Closed Angle Glaucoma

- Chronic angle closure
  - Portion of angle blocked
  - Develops scarring
  - Over time angle progressively more closed
  - Intraocular pressure not as high
  - Fewer symptoms (pain, etc.)
  - Delayed presentation
  - More damage to the optic nerve
  - Diagnosis made when peripheral vision loss occurs

Open Angle Glaucoma

- Chronic → most patients have this form
- No symptoms until loss of eyesight occurs
  - Peripheral then central
- Overproduction fluid or decreased drainage
- Angle for drainage of fluid is "open"
- Too much fluid or too little drainage
- Chronic drug therapy

Open Angle Glaucoma

- Associations
  - Age
  - Family history
  - African-American race

Open Angle Glaucoma

- Primary
  - Cause unclear
- Secondary
  - Uveitis
  - Trauma
  - Steroids
  - Retinopathy

Disc Cupping

Healthy Optic Nerve   Optic Nerve in Eye with Glaucoma

Image courtesy of GLAUCOMA RESEARCH FOUNDATION

Chronic Glaucoma Drugs

- M3 agonists
  - Contract ciliary muscle
- α2 agonists
  - Block ciliary epithelium from releasing aqueous
- β blockers
  - Block ciliary epithelium from releasing aqueous
- Prostaglandin analogues
  - Vasodilate the Canals of Schlemm: increase outflow
- Carbonic anhydrase inhibitors
  - Decrease synthesis of aqueous

Parasympathomimetics

- Carbachol, pilocarpine
- Muscarinic agonists
- Contract ciliary muscle
- Opens trabecular meshwork
- More drainage

Alpha Agonists

- Apraclonidine, Brimonidine
- Decrease aqueous production
- Can have (<15%) ocular side effects
  - Blurry vision
  - Ocular hyperemia
  - Foreign body sensation
  - Itchy eyes

Beta Blockers

- Timolol, betaxolol, carteolol
- ↓ aqueous humor production by ciliary epithelium

Prostaglandin analogues

- Bimatoprost, latanoprost, tafluprost, travoprost
- More drainage/outflow
- Will darken iris

Carbonic anhydrase inhibitors

- Acetazolamide (oral)
- Diuretic
- Less fluid production by ciliary epithelium

Epinephrine

- Mixed alpha-beta agonist
- Early effect: ↑aqueous humor (beta effect)
- Later effect: Vasoconstriction ciliary body
  - ↓production aqueous humor
- Never give in closed angle glaucoma
  - Dilates pupil
  - Worsens angle closure

General Anesthetics

Jason Ryan, MD, MPH

Anesthetic

- Drugs that produce:
  - Analgesia
  - Loss of consciousness
  - Amnesia
  - Muscle relaxation

Types of Anesthesia Drugs

- Inhaled anesthetics
- Intravenous anesthetics
- Local anesthetics
- Neuromuscular blocking agents

Inhaled Anesthetic Principles

- Special properties determine effectiveness
- Solubility of gas for blood determines onset/offset
- Solubility of gas for lipids determines potency

Blood Solubility
Inhaled Anesthetics

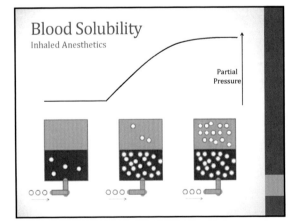

Partial Pressure

Blood Solubility
Inhaled Anesthetics

- Molecules dissolved in blood: No anesthetic effect
- Molecules NOT dissolved: Anesthetic effect
- Need to saturate blood to generate partial pressure
- So MORE solubility in blood = LONGER to take effect

Blood Solubility
Inhaled Anesthetics

Alveolar Gas ⟶ Saturated Blood ⟶ Brain Effect ⟶ Sedation

Blood Solubility
Inhaled Anesthetics

- Higher solubility
  - Higher tendency to stay in blood
  - Less likely to leave blood for brain
  - Longer time to saturate blood
  - SLOWER induction time (also washout time)
- Low solubility
  - Quickly saturate blood
  - Quickly exert effects on brain
  - SHORTER induction time (also washout time)

Blood Solubility
Inhaled Anesthetics

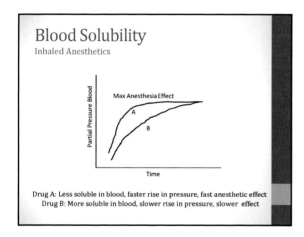

Drug A: Less soluble in blood, faster rise in pressure, fast anesthetic effect
Drug B: More soluble in blood, slower rise in pressure, slower effect

Blood Solubility
Inhaled Anesthetics

- Blood/gas partition coefficient
  - Isoflurane: 1.4
  - [blood]1.4 > [alveoli]

Blood Solubility
Inhaled Anesthetics

Gas	PC
Halothane	2.3
Isoflurane	1.4
Sevoflurane	0.69
Nitrous Oxide	0.47
Desflurane	0.42

Halothane → SLOW induction (like to stay in blood)
Nitric Oxide → FAST induction (quickly leaves blood)

Lipid Solubility
Inhaled Anesthetics

- Affinity of gas for a lipids
- Oil/gas partition coefficient
- ↑lipid affinity = more potent (Meyer-Overton rule)

Gas	PC
Halothane	224
Enflurane	99
Isoflurane	98
Sevoflurane	47
Desflurane	28
Nitrous Oxide	<10

Inhaled Anesthetic Principles

- Minimum alveolar concentration
  - Concentration of anesthetic that prevents movement in 50 percent of subjects in response to pain
- Low MAC = High potency
- MAC changes with age
  - Lower in elderly
- MAC related to lipid solubility (not blood!!)

$$\text{Lipid Solubility} = \frac{1}{MAC}$$

Inhaled Anesthetics Summary

- Onset of action
  - Blood:gas partition coefficient (↑higher = slower)
  - Solubility in blood (↑higher = slower)
- Potency
  - Oil/gas partition coefficient (↑higher = more potent)
  - MAC (↓lower = more potent)

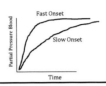

Inhaled Anesthetics

- Desflurane
- Sevoflurane
- Halothane
- Enflurane
- Isoflurane
- Methoxyflurane
- Nitrous oxide

Common Effects

- Myocardial depression
  - ↓CO
- Respiratory depression
- Nausea and vomiting
- ↑ cerebral blood flow
  - Cerebral vasodilation
  - Blood flow goes up
  - ICP goes up
- Decreased GFR

Special Side Effects

- Halothane – Hepatotoxicity & malignant hyperthermia
  - Liver tox: Rare, life-threatening
  - Massive necrosis, increased AST/ALT
- Methoxyflurane – Nephrotoxicity
  - Renal-toxic metabolite
- Enflurane – Seizures
  - Lowers seizure threshold

Malignant Hyperthermia

- Rare, dangerous reaction: halothane, succinylcholine
- Fever, muscle rigidity after surgery
- Tachycardia, hypertension
- Muscle damage: ↑K, CK
- Cause: ryanodine receptor sarcoplasmic reticulum
  - Ca channel in SR of muscle cells
  - Abnormal in patients who get MH (autosomal dominant)
  - Dumps calcium
  - Ca → consumption of ATP for SR reuptake
  - ATP consumption → heat → tissue damage
- Treat with dantrolene (muscle relaxant)

Nitrous Oxide

- Diffuses rapidly into air spaces
- Will increase volume
- Cannot use:
  - Pneumothorax
  - Abdominal distention
- 50% NO → doubling of cavity size

Intravenous Anesthetics

- Barbiturates
- Benzodiazepines
- Opioids
- Etomidate
- Ketamine
- Propofol

Barbiturates

- Thiopental (Pentothal)
- Binding to GABA-receptor
  - Different mechanism from benzodiazepines
- High potency from high lipid solubility
- Rapid onset
  - Rapid entry into brain
- Ultra short acting
  - Rapid distribution to muscle and fat
- Myocardial/respiratory depression
- ↓ cerebral blood flow

Benzodiazepines
Midazolam, Lorazepam, Diazepam, Alprazolam

- Bind to GABA receptors
- ↑ frequency of GABA ion channel opening
- Low dose: anti-anxiety (anxiolytic)
- High dose: sedation, amnesia, anticonvulsant
- Cause cardio-respiratory depression
  - ↓BP
- Overdose: Flumazenil
- Midazolam (Versed): Short procedures (endoscopy)

Opioids
Morphine, Fentanyl, Hydromorphone

- Sedatives, analgesics
- No amnesia
- Act on opioid (mu) receptors in brain
- Side effects:
  - ↓respiratory drive
  - ↓BP
  - Nausea/vomiting
  - Ileus
  - Urinary retention
- Tolerance: Decreased effectiveness chronic use

Opioids Mechanism
Morphine, Fentanyl, Hydromorphone

- Mu receptors
- G-protein linked
- 2nd messengers not clearly understood
- Increase K efflux from cells
- This HYPERpolarizes → less pain transmission

143

Naloxone

- Opioid antidote
- Used for overdose
- Mu antagonist
- Competes with opioids, displaces from binding site
- Reverses effects within minutes
- Must be given IV → inactivated by liver if PO

Opioid Tolerance

- Effect wanes with chronic use
- Major problem with cancer pain
- Decreased effect on
  - Pain
  - Sedation
  - Nausea, vomiting
  - Respiratory depression
  - Cough suppression
  - Urinary retention
- No tolerance to constipation or miosis
  - These effects persist

Ketamine

- PCP derivative
- Antagonist of NMDA receptor (glutamate)
- "Dissociative" drug
  - Patient enters trancelike state
  - Analgesia and amnesia
  - Few respiratory or CV effects
- Can cause ↑BP ↑HR

Ketamine

- "Emergence Reactions"
  - Disorientation
  - Dreams, hallucinations
  - Can be frightening to patients
  - Co-administer midazolam to help

Etomidate

- Modulates GABA receptors
  - Blocks neuroexcitation
- Anesthesia but not analgesia
- Relatively hemodynamically neutral
  - Good for hypotensive patients
- Blocks cortisol synthesis
- Rapid sequence intubation

Propofol

- GABA modulator
- Sedation, amnesia
- Myocardial depression, hypotension

144

GABA Receptor Anesthetics

- Etomidate
- Propofol
- Benzodiazepines
- Barbiturates
- GABA is largely inhibitory
- These drugs activate receptor → sedation

Induction & Maintenance

- Induction – Put patient to sleep
  - Propofol, Etomidate, Ketamine
- Maintenance – Keep patient asleep
  - Propofol, sevoflurane, desflurane

Typical Open Heart Case

- Induction
  - Propofol, Midazolam
- Paralysis
  - Rocuronium
- Maintenance
  - Sevoflurane, fentanyl

Local Anesthetics

Jason Ryan, MD, MPH

Local Anesthetics

- Amides
  - Lidocaine
  - Mepivacaine
  - Bupivacaine
- Esters
  - Procaine
  - Cocaine
  - Benzocaine
  - Tetracaine

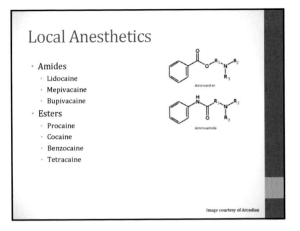

Image courtesy of Arcadian

Local Anesthetic

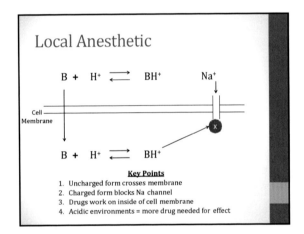

Key Points
1. Uncharged form crosses membrane
2. Charged form blocks Na channel
3. Drugs work on inside of cell membrane
4. Acidic environments = more drug needed for effect

Adding Epinephrine

- LA can be given with epinephrine
  - Causes vasoconstriction
  - Less bleeding
  - Less washout → more local effect

Differential Blockade

- Small fibers > large fibers
- Myelinated > unmyelinated

Order of Block	Fiber Type
1	Small, myelinated
2	Small, unmyelinated
3	Large, myelinated
4	Large, unmyelinated

Differential Blockade

- Different effects different senses
- Pain blocked first, pressure last

Order of Block	Fiber Type
1	Pain
2	Temp
3	Touch
4	Pressure

Local Anesthetics Uses

- Minor surgical procedures
- Epidural/spinal anesthesia

Local Anesthetics Side Effects

- CNS Stimulation
  - Initial (excitation):Talkativeness, anxiety, confusion, stuttering speech
  - Later: Drowsiness, coma
- Cardiovascular
  - Hypotension, arrhythmia, bradycardia, heart block
  - Cocaine is exception: hypertension, vasoconstriction
- Bupivacaine most cardiotoxic

Methemoglobinemia

- Iron in hemoglobin normally reduced (Fe^{2+})
- Certain drug oxidize iron to Fe^{3+}
- When Fe^{3+} is present → methemoglobin
- Fe^{3+} cannot bind oxygen
- Remaining Fe^{2+} cannot release to tissues
- Acquired methemoglobinemia from drugs
  - Local anesthetics (benzocaine)
  - Nitric oxide
  - Dapsone
- Treatment: methylene blue

Clinical Scenario

- Endoscopy patient
- Benzocaine spray used for throat analgesia
- Post procedure shortness of breath
- "Chocolate brown blood"
- O2 sat (pulse oximetry) = variable (80s-90s)
- PaO2 (blood gas) = normal
- Also premature babies given NO for pulmonary vasodilation

Neuromuscular Blockers

Jason Ryan, MD, MPH

Types of Anesthesia Drugs

- Inhaled anesthetics
- Intravenous anesthetics

- Neuromuscular blocking agents

Paralytics

- Succinylcholine
- Tubocurarine
- Atracurium
- Mivacurium
- Pancuronium
- Vecuronium
- Rocuronium

Succinylcholine

- Different from all other paralytics
- DEPOLARIZING neuromuscular blocker
- Basically two ACh molecules joined together
- Strong ACh (nicotinic) receptor agonist
- Sustained depolarization
- Prevent muscle contraction

Succinylcholine

- Two phases to depolarizing block
- Phase 1
  - Depolarizing phase
  - Muscle fasciculations occur
- Phase 2
  - Desensitizing phase
  - Depolarization has occurred
  - Muscle no longer reacts to ACh

Succinylcholine – Phase 1

- Na channels open and then close - become inactivated
- Membrane potential must reset
- Normally rapid as Ach hydrolysed by AChE
- Succinylcholine NOT metabolized by AChE
- Prolonged activation of ACh receptors occurs

Succinylcholine – Phase 2

- Desensitizing phase
- Normally ACh washed out quickly – no desensitization
- Longer depolarization (succ) → desensitization

Succinylcholine

- Fast acting
- Rapid washout
- No reversal
- Main side effect is ↑K
  - Caution in burn patients, dialysis patients
- Malignant Hyperthermia

Malignant Hyperthermia

- Rare, dangerous reaction: halothane, succinylcholine
- High fever, muscle rigidity after surgery
- Tachycardia, hypertension
- Muscle damage: ↑K, CK
- Cause: ryanodine receptor sarcoplasmic reticulum
  - Ca channel in SR of muscle cells
  - Abnormal in patients who get MH (autosomal dominant)
  - Dumps calcium
  - Ca → consumption of ATP for SR reuptake
  - ATP consumption → heat → tissue damage
- Treat with dantrolene (muscle relaxant)

Non-depolarizing NMBA
Tubocurarine, Atracurium, Mivacurium, Pancuronium, Vecuronium, Rocuronium

- Competitive antagonists
- Compete with ACh for nicotinic receptors
- Produce paralysis
- Many cause marked histamine release
  - Hypotension → compensatory tachycardia
- Can be reversed by flooding synapse with ACh
- This is done by inhibiting AChE

AChE Inhibitors
Reversal of non-depolarizing neuromuscular blockers

- Physostigmine
- Neostigmine
- Pyridostigmine
- Edrophonium

ICU Weakness

- Common after prolonged ICU treatment
- May be associated with NMBA

Assessing Neuromuscular Blockade

- Peripheral nerve stimulator
- Train of 4 impulses

Train of 4

- Used to assess neuromuscular blockade in patients under anesthesia
- 4 electrical stimulations to nerve (i.e. ulnar)
- Goal usually 1/4 or 2/4

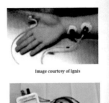

Image courtesy of Ignis

Image courtesy of Paunami

Rapid Sequence Intubation

- Standard practice for emergent intubation
- Renders patient sedated and flaccid
- Induction: Etomidate
  - Sometimes ketamine, benzos
- Paralysis: Succinylcholine

Meningitis

Jason Ryan, MD, MPH

The Meninges

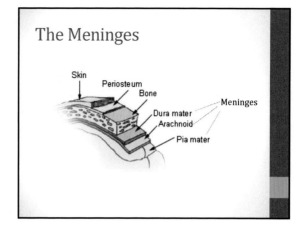

Skin
Periosteum
Bone
Meninges
Dura mater
Arachnoid
Pia mater

Meningitis

- Inflammation of the leptomeninges
- Usually infectious: viral, bacterial, fungal
- Rarely: cancer, sarcoid, inflammatory diseases

Symptoms

- Fever, headache, photophobia
- Nuchal rigidity
  - Nape = back of neck
  - Nuchal = related to nape
  - Nuchal rigidity = hurts to move back of neck

Symptoms

- Kernig sign
  - Thigh bent at hip with knee at 90 degrees
  - Subsequent extension of knee is painful (resistance)
- Brudzinski sign
  - Lye patient flat
  - Lift head off table
  - Involuntary lifting of legs
- Both signs of meningismus
  - Usually meningitis
  - Also subarachnoid hemorrhage

Diagnosis of Meningitis

- Suggestive signs & symptoms
- Spinal tap

Spinal Tap

Lumbar Puncture

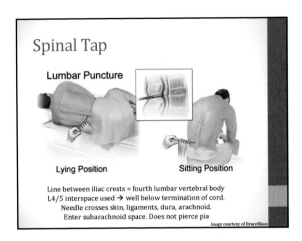

Lying Position   Sitting Position

Line between iliac crests = fourth lumbar vertebral body
L4/5 interspace used → well below termination of cord.
Needle crosses skin, ligaments, dura, arachnoid.
Enter subarachnoid space. Does not pierce pia

Image courtesy of BruceBlaus

Opening Pressure

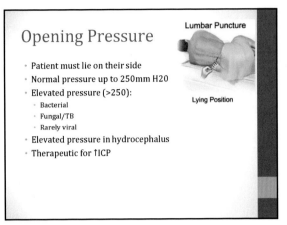

- Patient must lie on their side
- Normal pressure up to 250mm H20
- Elevated pressure (>250):
  - Bacterial
  - Fungal/TB
  - Rarely viral
- Elevated pressure in hydrocephalus
- Therapeutic for ↑ICP

Complications of Meningitis

- Death
- Hydrocephalus
- Hearing loss
- Seizures
- Most from bacterial meningitis

Selecting Treatment

- Antibiotics
- Culture takes days
- Cannot wait for culture to drive choice of drug
- Choose drugs based on:
  - Patient age, co-morbidities
  - Spinal fluid cell types, protein, glucose

Spinal Fluid Testing

- Cells
- Protein
- Glucose
- Culture

CSF Meningitis Findings

	Cells	Protein	Glucose
Bacterial	↑PMNs	↑	↓
Viral	↑lymphocytes	Normal or ↑	Normal
Fungal/TB	↑lymphocytes	↑	↓

Normal CSF

- Clear
- 0-5 lymphocytes
- <45mg/dl protein
- >45mg/dl glucose
  - About 2/3 of blood glucose (80-120)

Meningitis Antibiotics

- Ceftriaxone
- Vancomycin
- Ampicillin
- Gentamycin
- All have good CSF penetration

Causes of Meningitis

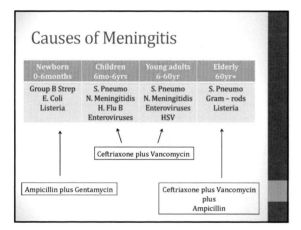

Newborn 0-6months	Children 6mo-6yrs	Young adults 6-60yr	Elderly 60yr+
Group B Strep E. Coli Listeria	S. Pneumo N. Meningitidis H. Flu B Enteroviruses	S. Pneumo N. Meningitidis Enteroviruses HSV	S. Pneumo Gram – rods Listeria

Ceftriaxone plus Vancomycin

Ampicillin plus Gentamycin

Ceftriaxone plus Vancomycin plus Ampicillin

Streptococcus Pneumoniae

- Most common cause meningitis all ages
- Lancet-shaped, gram positive cocci in pairs
- Can follow strep respiratory infection
- Increased risk
  - Asplenic patients
  - Sickle cell
  - Alcoholics
- Also causes otitis media (kids), pneumonia, sinusitis

Neisseria Meningitidis

- Gram negative cocci in pairs (diplococci)
- Transmitted by respiratory droplets
- Enters pharynx then bloodstream then CSF
- Many asymptomatic carriers
- Polysaccharide capsule prevents phagocytosis
- Lipooligosaccharide (LOS) outer membrane
  - Like LPS on gram negative rods
  - Endotoxin → many toxic effects on body
  - Activates severe inflammatory response

Neisseria Meningitidis

- Bacteremia can complicate meningitis
- Meningococcemia
- Sepsis: fevers, chills, tachycardia
- Purpuric rash
- DIC
- Waterhouse-Friderichsen syndrome
  - Adrenal destruction from meningococcemia
- Life-threatening

Neisseria Meningitidis

- Can cause outbreaks
  - Dorms, barracks
- Can infect young, healthy people
  - College students in dorms
- Infected patients need droplet precautions
- Close contracts receive prophylaxis
  - Rifampin
  - Also Ceftriaxone or Ciprofloxacin
- Vaccine available
  - Contains capsular polysaccharides → anti-capsule antibodies
  - Only used in high risk groups

Haemophilus Influenzae

- Small, gram negative rod (coccobacillus)
- Enters pharynx then lymphatics then CSF

H. Influenza Vaccine

- HIB once most common cause bacterial meningitis
- Hib conjugate vaccines given in infancy
- H. Flu meningitis almost always occurs in unimmunized children
  - May immigrate from other countries without vaccination

Listeria

- Gram positive rod
- Facultative intracellular organism
- "Tumbling motility"
- Multiplies in cells with poor cell-mediated immunity
  - Neonates, HIV, organ transplant
- In adults, often from contaminated food
  - Undercooked meat, unwashed vegetables
  - Unpasteurized cheese/milk
  - Likes cold temperatures
- In neonates, transplacental or vaginal transmission

Group B Strep

- Strep Agalactiae
- Gram positive cocci in chains
  - Catalase negative
  - Beta hemolytic bacteria
  - CAMP test positive
- Most common cause meningitis in newborns
  - Transmitted when baby passes through birth canal
  - Ampicillin during labor can prevent
- May not have classic symptoms
  - Hypotonia, weak sucking reflex
  - Bulging fontanels, sunken eyes
  - Poor feeding

E. Coli

- 2nd most common meningitis cause neonates
- Motile, gram-negative bacillus (rod)
- Some strains have K-1 capsular antigen
  - Inhibits complements, other immune responses
  - Allows bacteria to evade host immunity
- Grows on:
  - Blood agar
  - MacConkey agar
  - Eosin methylene blue agar

Viral Meningitis

- Old name: "aseptic"
  - Evidence of meningitis without bacteria
- Usually enteroviruses
  - Coxsackievirus, echovirus, poliovirus
- Self-limited
- Supportive care – no specific treatment
- All single stranded RNA viruses
- Fecal-oral transmission

Viral Meningitis

- Rare causes
  - HSV
  - HIV
  - West Nile virus
  - Varicella Zoster virus

Herpes Virus

- HSV-1
  - Oral herpes
  - Eye infections (keratoconjunctivitis)
  - Encephalitis - Loves to infect the TEMPORAL lobe
- HSV-2
  - Genital herpes
  - 13 to 36% primary genital herpes pts have clinical findings of meningitis (headache, photophobia and meningismus)
  - Genital lesions in 85% patients with HSV-2 meningitis
- Treatment: acyclovir, valacyclovir, famciclovir

Viral Meningitis

- Usually no specific virus testing
- If HIV suspected
  - Blood testing for HIV RNA and HIV antibody
- If HSV suspected anti-virals can be given
- Other viruses tested only special circumstances

TB Meningitis

- M. tuberculosis infection of the meninges
- CSF lymphocytes
- High protein, low glucose
- Need multiple CSF samples for culture
- Acid-fast bacilli (AFB) sometimes seen in CSF
- Nucleic acid amplification tests (NAATs) used
  - Use polymerase chain reaction (PCR) techniques

Encephalitis

- Encephalitis = brain inflammation
- Must make sure meningitis patients don't have:
  - Altered mental status
  - Motor or sensory deficits
  - Altered behavior and personality changes
  - Speech/movement disorders
- If these are present, HSV-1 is common cause

Encephalitis
Other (rare) causes

- Varicella-zoster (chickenpox, shingles)
- Mosquito viruses
  - St. Louis encephalitis virus
  - Eastern/western equine
  - West Nile
  - California encephalitis

Encephalitis
Other (rare) causes

- Lassa fever encephalitis
  - Spread by mice
  - Hemorrhagic virus like Ebola (many other symptoms)
- Measles
- Naegleria fowleri (protozoa)
- HIV Encephalitis

Seizures

Jason Ryan, MD, MPH

What is a seizure

- Sudden alteration in behavior
- Due to transient brain pathology

Seizure symptoms

- Loss of consciousness
- Abnormal motor activity
- Abnormal sensation
- Range
  - Mild: Loss of awareness (absence)
  - Severe: Tonic-clonic

Seizure Causes

- Many people have 1 seizure
- Often "provoked"
  - Fever (children)
  - Lack of sleep
  - Drugs, alcohol
  - Hypoglycemia
- Other causes more serious: tumors, strokes
- Multiple, unprovoked seizures is epilepsy

Seizure Causes by Age Group

Children	Adults	Elderly
Genetic	Tumors	Stroke
Fever	Trauma	Tumor
Trauma	Stroke	Trauma
Congenital	Infection	Metabolic
Metabolic		Infection

Genetic: Juvenile myoclonic epilepsy
Metabolic: Hyponatremia, hypernatremia, hypoMg, hypoCa
Infection: Meningoencephalitis

Seizure Workup

- Blood work
- EKG (cardiac syncope)
- EEG
- Brain imaging (CT or MRI)
- Sometimes lumbar puncture (LP)

EEG
Electroencephalogram

- Records voltage changes in brain
- Different leads
  - Frontal, parietal, occipital
- Characteristic patterns

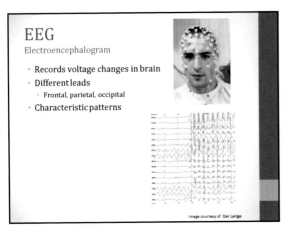

Image courtesy of Der Lange

Seizure Types

- Partial – One discrete part of brain
  - Simple partial – No alteration consciousness
  - Complex partial – Alteration consciousness
- Generalized – Entire brain effected
  - Absence "Petit mal"
  - Tonic-clonic "Grand mal"
  - Atonic "Drop seizure"
  - Myotonic
- Secondary generalized

Psychic Symptoms

- Can occur with partial seizures
- Higher cortical areas affected
- Dysphasia
- Feelings of familiarity ("deja-vu")
- Distortions of time
- Fear
- Hallucinations

Autonomic Symptoms

- Epigastric "rising" sensation
  - Common aura with medial temporal lobe epilepsy
- Sweating
- Piloerection
- Pupillary changes

Auras

- Warning before major seizure
- Auras = simple, partial seizures
- Seizure affects enough brain to cause symptoms
- Not enough to interfere with consciousness
- Symptoms depend on area of brain
  - Occipital lobe: flashing lights
  - Motor cortex: muscle jerking (Jacksonian Seizure)

Post-ictal State

- Transition period seizure → normal state
- Period of brain recovery
- Confusion, lack of alertness
- Focal neurologic deficits may present
- Variable time, minutes to hours

Partial Seizures

- Most common site: temporal lobe
- Mesial temporal sclerosis
  - Also called hippocampal sclerosis
  - Neuronal loss in hippocampus
- Often bilateral but one side>other
- Can diagnose by MRI

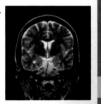

Juvenile Myoclonic Epilepsy

- Absence, myoclonic, and grand mal
- Common in children
- Absence seizures first (~5 years of age)
- Myoclonic seizures later (~15 years)
- Grand mal seizures soon after
- Hallmark:
  - Myoclonic jerks on awakening from sleep
  - Shock-like, irregular movements of both arms

Childhood Absence Epilepsy

- Sudden impairment of consciousness
- No change in body/motor tone
- Last few seconds
- Usually remits by puberty
- Classic EEG finding: 2.5 - 5 Hertz spike wave activity superimposed on normal background EEG
- No post-ictal confusion
- Ethosuximide is first line treatment
  - Blocks thalamic T-type Ca++ channels

Febrile Seizures

- Common: 2-4% children <5 years old
- Child loses consciousness, shakes
- Children at risk for more febrile seizures
- Overall prognosis generally good
- This is NOT considered epilepsy

Eclampsia

- Pregnancy related condition
- 20weeks to 6weeks post-partum
- Hypertension, proteinuria, edema = Preeclampsia
- Eclampsia = preeclampsia + seizures
- Treatment: MgSO4

Seizure Treatment Principles

- Breaking seizures
  - Status epilepticus
  - Continuous seizure >30min
  - Or seizure that recurs <30min
  - Medical emergency
  - Arrhythmias, lactic acidosis, hypertension
- Preventing seizures

Breaking Seizures

- First line treatment is benzodiazepines
  - Rapid acting
- Lorazepam drug of choice
- Also often administer:
  - Phenytoin (PO) or fosphenytoin (IV)
  - Prevent recurrent seizures
- If still seizing after benzo/phenytoin → phenobarbital
- Often will then give general anesthesia and intubuate

Preventing Seizures

Na Inactivators
- Phenytoin
- Carbamazepine
- Lamotrigine
- Valproic Acid

GABA Activators
- Phenobarbital
- Tiagabine
- Vigabatrin
- Valproic Acid

Other Mechanisms
- Gabapentin
- Topiramate
- Ethosuximide
- Levetiracetam
- Primidone

Niche Drugs

- Status Epilepticus
  - Benzodiazepines
- Absence seizures
  - Ethosuximide

Teratogenicity

- All AEDs carry risk if taken during pregnancy
- Valproic Acid carries the greatest risk
  - Most teratogenic
  - 1-3% chance of neural tube defects

Carbamazepine

- Inactivates Na channels
- Useful for partial and generalized seizures
- Also: bipolar disorder, trigeminal neuralgia
- Many, many side effects
- Diplopia, ataxia
- Low blood counts
  - Agranulocytosis
  - Aplastic anemia

Carbamazepine

- Bone marrow suppression
  - Anemia, low WBC, low platelets
  - Monitor CBC
- Liver toxicity
  - Monitor LFTs
- SIADH (low Na level)
- Stevens-Johnson syndrome
- Drug blood levels monitored

Stevens Johnson Syndrome

- Rare, life-threatening skin condition
- Malaise and fever (URI Sx)
- Extensive skin lesions
- Skin necrosis and sloughing
- Can be triggered by meds, often AEDs
  - Carbamazepine
  - Ethosuximide
  - Phenytoin
  - Lamotrigine

Ethosuximide

- Blocks thalamic T-type Ca++ channels
- Drug of choice: childhood absence seizures
- Can cause SJS
- Other side effects
  - Nausea/vomiting
  - Sleep disruption
  - Fatigue, Hyperactivity

Phenobarbital

- Barbiturate
- Binding to GABA-receptor
  - Different mechanism from benzodiazepines
  - Increase duration channel is open
  - More Cl- flux
  - Less firing
- Myocardial/respiratory depression
- CNS depression, worse with EtOH
- Contraindicated in porphyria
- Induces P450 enzyme system

Cytochrome P450

- Intracellular enzymes
- Metabolize many drugs
- If inhibited → drug levels rise
- If induced → drug levels fall
- AEDs that induce CYP450
  - Carbamazepine
  - Phenobarbital
  - Phenytoin

Cytochrome P450

- Inhibitors are more dangerous
  - Can cause drug levels to rise
  - Cyclosporine, some macrolides, azole antifungals
- Luckily, many P450 metabolized drugs rarely used
  - Theophylline, Cisapride, Terfenadine
- Some clinically relevant possibilities
  - Some statins + Inhibitor → Rhabdo
  - Warfarin

P450 Drugs
Some Examples

Inducers	Inhibitors
Chronic EtOH	Isoniazid
Rifampin	Erythromycin
Phenobarbital	Cimetidine
Carbamazepine	Azoles
Griseofulvin	Grapefruit juice
Phenytoin	Ritonavir (HIV)

Phenytoin

- Inactivates Na channels
- Very useful tonic-clonic seizures
- Gingival hyperplasia, hair growth
- Rash
- Folic acid depletion (supplement)
- Decreased bone density
- Long term use: nystagmus, diplopia, ataxia
- Teratogenic
- Monitor blood levels

Gingival Hyperplasia

Image courtesy of Lesion

Phenytoin

- Dose-dependent hepatic metabolism
- Low dose → small ↑ blood levels
- High dose → enzymes saturated → rapid ↑ levels
- Induces and is metabolized by P450
- Co-admin with P450 drugs alters levels

Image courtesy of Lesion

Valproic Acid

- Na and GABA effects
  - ↑synthesis, ↓breakdown GABA
- Also a mood stabilizer (bipolar disorder, acute mania)
- BAD for pregnancy
  - Associated with spina bifida
- Nausea / vomiting
- Hepatotoxic – Check LFTs
- Tremor, weight gain

Levetiracetam

- Exact mechanism unknown
- Useful for many types of seizures
- Blood levels can be monitored
- Drug titrated to clinical effect
- Well tolerated: few important/serious side effects

Other AEDs

- Lamotrigine
  - Na channel drug
  - SJS – Discontinue if rash develops, especially kids
- Gabapentin
  - Affects Ca channels
  - Sedation, ataxia

Other AEDs

- Topiramate
  - Na and GABA effects
  - Mental dulling, sedation
  - Weight loss
  - Kidney stones
- Primidone
  - Exact mechanism not clear
  - Metabolized to phenobarbital
  - Also can be used for essential tremor

Neuroembryology

Jason Ryan, MD, MPH

Germ Layers

- Mesoderm
  - CV system, muscles, bone
- Endoderm
  - Liver, lungs, GI tract
- Ectoderm (Most CNS)
  - Surface ectoderm: ant pituitary, lens, cornea
  - Neural tube: brain, spinal cord, post pituitary, retina
  - Neural crest: Autonomic, sensory nerves, skull

Neural Tube Development

- Developmental process starts with notochord
- Secretes signal molecules (Sonic Hedgehog protein)
- Induces overlying ectoderm → neuroectoderm
- Neuroectoderm becomes neural plate
- Neural plate becomes neural tube
  - Also neural crest cells
- All occurs days 17-21 in embryo
- Notochord in adult: nucleus pulposus (IV discs)

Neural Tube Development

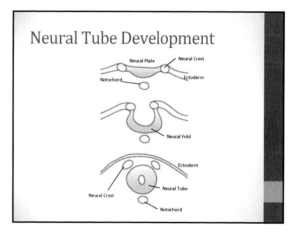

Nucleus Pulposus

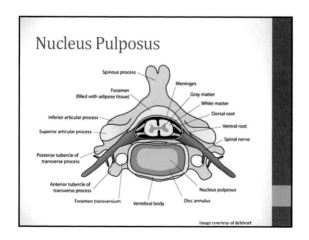

Alar and Basal Plates

- Alar is doral (posterior) → Sensory
- Basal is ventral (anterior) → Motor

Regional Brain Development

- Neural tube has bulges/swellings
- 3 primary vesicles (bulges)
  - Forebrain (prosencephalon)
  - Midbrain (mesencephalon)
  - Hindbrain (rhombencephalon)
- 5 secondary vesicles
  - Telencephalon
  - Diencephalon
  - Mesencephalon
  - Metencephalon
  - Myelencephalon

Regional Brain Development

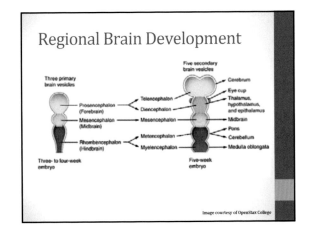

Image courtesy of OpenStax College

Neuro Congenital Defects

- Neural Tube Defects
  - Spina Bifida (caudal end of tube)
  - Anencephaly (rostral end)
  - Encephalocele
- Cephalic disorders
  - Holoprosencephaly
- Posterior Fossa Defects
  - Chiari malformations
  - Dandy Walker

Neural Tube Defects

- Neuropores fail to fuse in 4th week
  - Neuropore = opening of neural tube
  - Rostral neuropore at head, Caudal at tail
- Spina Bifida
  - Caudal neuropore fails to close posteriorly
  - Bones do not close around spinal cord/meninges
- Anencephaly ("without head")
  - Rostral neuropore fails to close anteriorly
  - Absence of major portions brain/skull

Neural Tube Defect Risks

- ↓folic acid intake
- Type I diabetes
- Obesity
- Valproic acid and/or carbamazepine

Spina Bifida

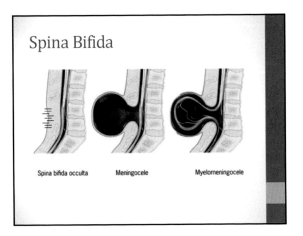

Spina bifida occulta   Meningocele   Myelomeningocele

Spina Bifida

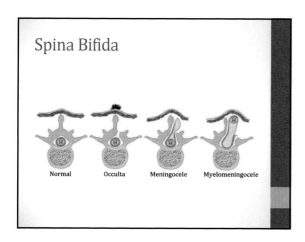

Normal   Occulta   Meningocele   Myelomeningocele

Spina Bifida

- Defects can be detected in utero
- Surgery can repair the defect
  - Sometimes in utero, often after birth
- Permanent neuro deficits often result
  - Leg weakness or paralysis (wheelchair)
  - Bowel/bladder problems

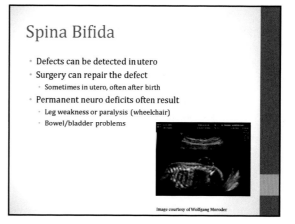

Image courtesy of Wolfgang Moroder

Anencephaly

- Forebrain/brainstem exposed in utero
- Fail to develop
- Not compatible with life
- Stillbirth or death shortly after birth
- Ultrasound:
  - Open calvaria
  - Frog-like appearance of fetus
- Mother will have polyhydramnios
  - Baby can't swallow amniotic fluid normally

Encephalocele

- Brain or meninges herniate through skull defect
- Least common NTD
- Most common site: occipital bone

Alpha Fetal Protein

- Fetal specific globulin
- Made by fetal yolk sac, fetal organs
- Function unknown
- Excreted by fetal kidneys
- 16 to 18 weeks → measure maternal serum level
- If high, MAY indicated NTD
  - Interpretation complex
- Follow-up tests
  - Amniotic fluid AFP (requires amniocentesis)
  - Amniotic fluid acetylcholinesterase (AChE)
  - If both elevated, strongly suggests NTD

Prenatal Screening

- Neural tube defect screening
  - Ultrasound
  - Maternal blood level Alpha Fetal Protein (AFP)
- Screening also done for Down Syndrome
  - Nuchal translucency by ultrasound
  - Serum markers
- "Triple screen"
  - AFP
  - Estradiol
  - HCG

Holoprosencephaly

- Cephalic malformation
- Failure of cleavage of prosencephalon
- Left/right hemispheres fail to separate
- Usually happens during weeks 5-6
- Failure of signaling molecules
  - Sonic hedgehog implicated
- Key findings are facial abnormalities:
  - Cleft lip/palate
  - Cyclopia
- Associations: trisomy 13 (Patau syndrome), trisomy 18 (Edward's syndrome), Fetal alcohol syndrome

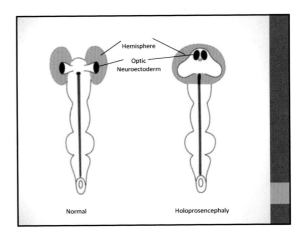

Normal   Holoprosencephaly

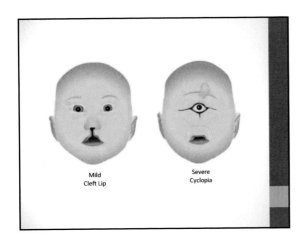

Mild
Cleft Lip

Severe
Cyclopia

Chiari Malformations

- Anatomic anomalies of cerebellum
- Group of congenital disorders
  - Chiari I through IV
- Downward displacement of the cerebellum

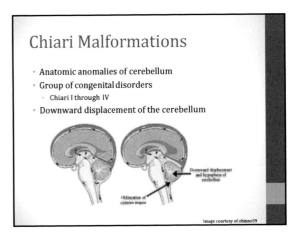

Image courtesy of obinno59

Chiari I Malformation

- Abnormal shape of cerebellar tonsils
  - Tonsils = small rounded structure bottom of cerebellum
- Tonsils displaced below foramen magnum
- Associated with Syringomyelia

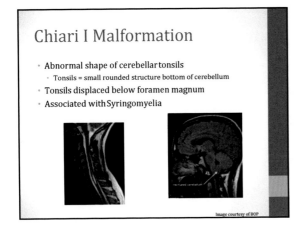

Image courtesy of BOP

Chiari I Malformation

- Usually no symptoms until adolescence/adulthood
  - Mean age 18 years
- Headaches
  - Due to meningeal irritation
  - Worse with cough: "cough headache"
- Other symptoms
  - Cerebellar dysfunction (ataxia)
  - Cranial nerve dysfunction (brainstem compression)

Chiari II Malformation
Arnold-Chiari Malformation

- Downward displacement cerebellar vermis & tonsils
- Brainstem malformation
  - Beaked midbrain on neuroimaging
- Spinal myelomeningocele
  - Usually detected prenatal/birth

Chiari II Malformation
Arnold-Chiari Malformation

- Blockage of aqueduct
- Hydrocephalus
- Myelomeningocele → paralysis below defect
- Hydrocephalus in infants
  - Large head circumference on growth curves
  - Anterior fontanelle distended
  - Sutures widely split
  - Abnormal percussion: "cracked pot" sound or Macewen's sign

Dandy Walker Malformation

- Developmental anomaly of the fourth ventricle
- Often detected by ultrasound in utero
- Hypoplasia or agenesis of cerebellar vermis
- Cerebellar hemispheres often flattened
  - Separated by "Dandy-Walker cyst"
- Cysts of 4th ventricle → hydrocephalus
- Many, many associated symptoms/conditions
- Affected children
  - Hydrocephalus
  - Delayed development
  - Motor dysfunction (crawling, walking)

Dandy Walker Malformation

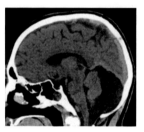

Delirium & Dementia

Jason Ryan, MD, MPH

Dementia vs. Delirium

- Dementia
  - Chronic, progressive cognitive decline
  - Usually irreversible
- Delirium
  - Acute
  - Waxing/waning
  - Usually reversible

Delirium

- Loss of focus/attention
- Disorganized thinking
- Hallucinations (often visual)
- Sleep-wake disturbance
  - Up at night
  - Sleeping during day

Delirium Causes

- Usually secondary to another cause
- Infection
- Alcohol
- Withdrawal
- Dementia patient in unknown setting
  - Classic scenario: demented patient with PNA
- Most common reason AMS in hospital

EEG
Electroencephalogram

- Records voltage changes in brain
- Different leads
  - Frontal, parietal, occipital
- Characteristic patterns
- NORMAL in dementia
- ABNORMAL in delirium

Image courtesy of Der Lange

Delirium Treatment

- Fix underlying cause
  - Treat infection, withdrawal, etc.
  - Maintain O2 levels
  - Treat pain
  - Hydrate
- Calm, quiet environment
- Drugs
  - Haloperidol (vitamin H)

168

Haloperidol
Trifluoperazine, fluphenazine, thioridazine, chlorpromazine

- Neuroleptics
  - Main effect is to block CNS dopamine (D2) receptors
  - Also block Ach (M), α1, histamine
- Uses
  - Schizophrenia
  - Psychosis
  - Mania

Haloperidol
Trifluoperazine, fluphenazine, thioridazine, chlorpromazine

- High potency agents
  - Haloperidol, trifluoperazine, fluphenazine
  - More neurologic side effects
  - Extrapyramidal side effects
- Low potency agents
  - Thioridazine, chlorpromazine
  - More non-neurologic side effects

Pyramidal vs. Extrapyramidal

- Pyramidal system
  - Corticospinal tract
  - Run in pyramids of medulla
  - Damage → weakness
- Extrapyramidal system
  - Basal ganglia nuclei and associated tracts
  - Rubrospinal, tectospinal, others
  - Modulation of movement
  - Damage → movement disorders

EPS Side Effects Haloperidol

- Exact mechanism unknown
- Response to dopamine receptor blockade
- Four movement side effects
  - Dystonia
  - Akathisia
  - Bradykinesia
  - Tardive dyskinesia

EPS Side Effects Haloperidol

- Dystonia – acute, within hours/days
  - Involuntary contraction of muscles
  - Spasms, stiffness
  - Treatment: benztropine
- Akathisia - days
  - Restlessness, urge to move
  - Sometimes misdiagnosed as worsening agitation
  - Treatment: Lower dose, benzos, propranolol

EPS Side Effects Haloperidol

- Bradykinesia - weeks
  - "Drug-induced Parkinsonism"
  - Slow movements, like Parkinson's
  - Treatment: benztropine
- Tardive dyskinesia – months/years
  - Chorea
  - Smacking lips
  - Grimacing
  - Often irreversible! (stopping drug doesn't help!)

169

EPS Side Effects Haloperidol

- Common with high potency drugs
  - Haloperidol
  - Trifluoperazine
  - Fluphenazine
- Less common with low potency drugs
  - Thioridazine
  - Chlorpromazine

Other Haloperidol Side Effects

- Blocks dopamine
  - Hyperprolactinemia
  - Galactorrhea
- Blocks ACh muscarinic receptors
  - Dry mouth
  - Constipation
- Blocks α1 receptors
  - Hypotension
- Blocks H receptors
  - Sedation
- Qt prolongation

- More common with low potency agents
  - Thioridazine
  - Chlorpromazine

NMS
Neuroleptic Malignant Syndrome

- Rare, dangerous reaction to neuroleptics
- Very similar to malignant hyperthermia
  - Reaction to halothane, succinylcholine
  - Same treatment: dantrolene (muscle relaxant)
- Usually 7-10 days after treatment with haldol

NMS
Neuroleptic Malignant Syndrome

- Fever, rigid muscles
- Mental status changes (encephalopathy)
- Hypertension, tachycardia
  - Autonomic instability
- Elevated CK
- Myoglobinuria - acute renal failure from rhabdo
- Watch for fever, rigidity, confusion after Haldol
- Treatment:
  - Dantrolene (muscle relaxant)
  - Bromocriptine (dopamine agonist)

Dementia

- Gradual decline in cognition
- No change LOC
- Usually irreversible (unlike delirium)
- Memory deficits
- Impaired judgment
- Personality changes

Dementia

- Aphasia
  - Inability to communicate effectively
  - Forget words
  - Can't understand (may nod to pretend)
- Apraxia
  - Inability to do pre-programmed motor tasks
  - Can't do their job
  - Later: chewing, swallowing, walking
- Agnosia
  - Inability to correctly interpret senses
  - Can't recognize people
  - Can't interpret full bladder, pain

Mini Mental Status Exam

- Point system
- >=27 (out of 30) is normal
- Oriented to time, place
- Repeat three objects, remember them
- Serial 7s or spell WORLD backwards
- Name an object pointed out (agnosia)
- Repeat a phrase
- Draw an object shown

Dementia Causes

- Alzheimer's disease - 60% of cases
- Multi-infarct dementia (stroke) ~20% of cases
- Lewy body dementia
- Rare stuff
  - Pick's disease
  - NPH
  - Creutzfeldt-Jakob
  - HIV
  - Vitamin deficiencies
  - Wilson's disease

Alzheimer's Disease

- Most common cause dementia
- Degeneration of cortex
  - Contrast with basal ganglia in movement disorders
  - Generalized → no focal deficits
- Characterized by loss of ACh cortical activity
  - Deficiency of choline acetyltransferase
  - Prominent in basal nucleus of Meynert and hippocampus

Alzheimer's BioChem

Amyloid Precursor Protein (APP)
(on neurons)

| Apolipoprotein E (ApoE) Epsilon 2 Allele | | Apolipoprotein E (ApoE) Epsilon 4 Allele |

Beta Breakdown Product
(cleavage)

↓

Alpha-Beta (AB) Amyloid

↓ CNS Buildup

Alzheimer's

Amyloid

- Proteins in many diseases
- Extracellular deposits
- All stain with Congo red
- All have apple-green birefringence (polarized light)
- Disease process depends on where they are found
- Alzheimer's: Brain

Alzheimer's Disease

- Major risk factor is age
  - Disease of elderly
  - Sporadic
- Early disease
  - Down syndrome – APP on Chromosome 21
  - Familial Form: Presenilin 1 & 2 gene mutations

Alzheimer's Disease

- Other risk factors:
  - African American race
  - Family history
  - Obesity
  - Type II diabetes (insulin resistance)
  - HTN, Hyperlipidemia
  - Traumatic brain injury

Alzheimer's Brain

- Cortical atrophy
- Gyri narrow
- Sulci widen
- Hydrocephalus ex vacuo
  - Ventricles appear larger due to atrophy

Healthy Brain   Severe AD

Alzheimer's Path

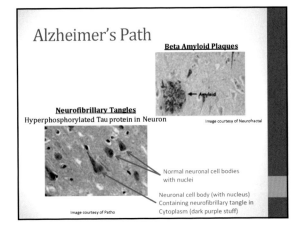

Beta Amyloid Plaques

← Amyloid

Image courtesy of Neurofractal

Neurofibrillary Tangles
Hyperphosphorylated Tau protein in Neuron

Normal neuronal cell bodies with nuclei

Neuronal cell body (with nucleus) Containing neurofibrillary tangle in Cytoplasm (dark purple stuff)

Image courtesy of Patho

Alzheimer's Symptoms

- Patient may not notice cognitive decline
- Often brought in by family member
- Diagnosis: clinical
- Confirmed at autopsy

Alzheimer's Drugs

- Memantine
  - NMDA receptor blocker
  - N-methyl-D-aspartate receptor (glutamate receptor)
  - Side Fx: Dizziness, confusion, hallucinations
- Donepezil, galantamine, rivastigmine
  - Inhibit acetylcholinesterase
  - Side Fx: Nausea, dizziness, insomnia
- Vitamin E
  - Believes to protect against oxidation

Multi-infarct Dementia

- Second most common cause
- Dementia after multiple strokes
- Vascular risk factors: HTN, ↑chol, smoking
- Stepwise progression of symptoms
- Treat risk factors

Lewy Body Dementia

- Lewy body: protein alpha-synuclein
- Found in basal ganglia in Parkinson's
- If found in cortex: LB dementia
- Triad
  - Dementia
  - Parkinson's symptoms
  - Hallucinations

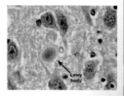

Image courtesy of Charles E. Driscoll, MD

Pick's Disease

- Rare cause of dementia
- Affects frontal and temporal lobes
  - Frontal: Change in personality, behavior
  - Temporal: Aphasia
- Path: Pick bodies
  - SPHERICAL tau proteins
  - Not tangles like AD

Creutzfeldt-Jakob

- "Spongiform encephalopathy"
- Intracellular vacuoles
- Caused by PrPSC prion
  - Sporadic mutation
  - Familial
  - Transmitted
- Mad Cow Disease

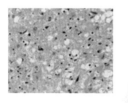

Creutzfeldt-Jakob

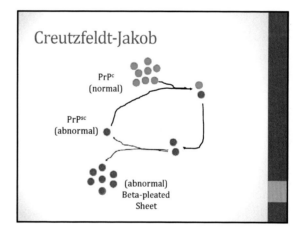

Creutzfeldt-Jakob

- Rapidly progressive dementia
- Death within a year
- Classic features
  - Ataxia
  - "Startle myoclonus"
  - Spike-wave complexes on EEG
- Diagnosis
  - Brain biopsy (gold standard)
  - Clinical criteria

Demyelinating Diseases

Jason Ryan, MD, MPH

Demyelinating Diseases

- Multiple Sclerosis
- Guillain-Barre syndrome
- Progressive multifocal leukoencephalopathy (PML)
- Postinfectious encephalomyelitis
- Charcot-Marie-Tooth disease
- Metachromatic leukodystrophy
- Krabbe's disease

Multiple Sclerosis

- Autoimmune demyelination CNS
- Brain and spinal cord
- White women in 20s & 30s is classic demographic
- Relapsing, remitting course (most commonly)
- Diverse neuro symptoms that come/go over time
- Fatigue is extremely common

Multiple Sclerosis

- Lymphocytes (T-cells) react to myelin antigens
- Myelin basic protein
- Interferon-gamma
- Recruit macrophages
- Type IV hypersensitivity reaction

Symptoms

- Any neuro symptom possible
- Few classic ones important to know
- Optic neuritis
  - Demyelination of optic nerve
  - Pain and loss of vision
- MLF syndrome (INO)
  - One eye cannot move medially on lateral gaze
- Bladder dysfunction
  - Spastic bladder
  - Overflow incontinence

MS Diagnosis

- MRI is gold standard
- Path: Periventricular plaques
  - Oligodendrocyte loss
  - Reactive gliosis
- CSF
  - High protein
  - Oligoclonal bands

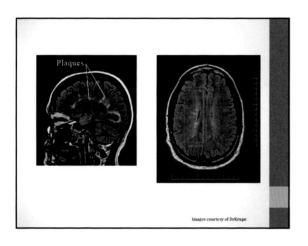

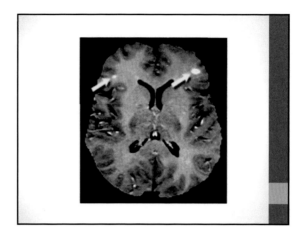

MS Treatment

- Rare patients do not require treatment
  - 1 or 2 lesions, no flairs
- Interferon (avonex, rebif, betaseron)
- Newer agents:
  - Natalizumab (Tysabri)
  - Dimethyl fumarate (Tecfidera)

Guillain-Barre syndrome

- Acute inflammatory demyelinating radiculopathy
- Schwann cells destroyed by immune system
- Ascending muscle weakness over days→weeks
  - Starts in legs
  - Spreads to other areas
  - Respiratory failure 10-30%
  - Facial muscle weakness >50%
- Sensory deficits occur (paresthesias) but mild
- Symptoms usually resolve over weeks to months

Peripheral Nerves

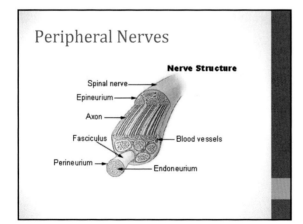

Guillain-Barre syndrome

- Autonomic dysfunction >70%
  - Tachycardia
  - Urinary retention
  - Hypertension/hypotension
  - Arrhythmias
  - Ileus
  - Loss of sweating
- Severe autonomic dysfunction can cause SCD

Guillain-Barre syndrome

- Often triggered by infection
- Classic agent: Campylobacter jejuni
  - Bloody diarrhea
- Classic agent: CMV
  - Usually asymptomatic infection
  - Detected by rise in CMV antibodies
  - Immunosuppressed patient (1-6months after xplant)
  - Febrile illness

Guillain-Barre syndrome

- CSF shows elevated protein level
- Normal CSF cell count

Guillain-Barre syndrome

- Treatment: Respiratory support
- Plasmapheresis
- IV immune globulins

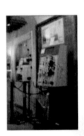

Image courtesy of Mr Vacchi

Progressive multifocal leukoencephalopathy (PML)

- Severe demyelinating disease of CNS
- Reactivation of a latent JC virus
- Demyelination: multiple white matter lesions imaging
- Destroys oligodendrocytes
- CD4 < 200 cells/mm3
- Causes slow onset encephalopathy
  - Altered mental status
  - Focal neuro defects (motor, gait, etc)
- Dx: JC Virus DNA in CSF or brain biopsy

Postinfectious encephalomyelitis

- Acute onset multifocal neurologic symptoms
- Often rapid deterioration → hospitalization
- Rare sequelae of infection or vaccinations
  - Mean 26 days after
  - Infections: Varicella or measles
  - Vaccines: Rabies, small pox
- Most common histopathology: perivenous infiltration
  - Lymphocytes, neutrophils, other cells
  - Inflammation/demyelination

Postinfectious encephalomyelitis

Images courtesy of Professor Yasser Metwally

176

Charcot-Marie-Tooth
Hereditary motor and sensory neuropathy (HMSN)

- Progressive hereditary peripheral nerve disorders
- Onset usually late childhood/adolescence
- Defective production nerve proteins or myelin
- Leg muscles (bilateral) become wasted
- Legs have characteristic stork-like contour
- Footdrop
- Foot deformities usually develop
- Upper extremities also affected (<lower)
- Falls, clumsiness

Charcot-Marie-Tooth
Hereditary motor and sensory neuropathy (HMSN)

- Progressive hereditary peripheral nerve disorders
- Onset usually late childhood/adolescence
- Defective production nerve proteins or myelin
- Leg muscles (bilateral) become wasted
- Legs have characteristic stork-like contour
- Footdrop
- Foot deformities usually develop
- Upper extremities also affected (<lower)
- Falls, clumsiness

Charcot-Marie-Tooth
Hereditary motor and sensory neuropathy (HMSN)

Pes cavus deformities

Claw Hands

Images courtesy of Dr. Sajida Khalid

Metachromatic leukodystrophy

- Lysosomal storage disease
- Rare, autosomal-recessive
  - Both parents must have mutation to pass on
- Progressive demyelination CNS, PNS
- Arylsulfatase A deficiency
- Buildup of sulfatides → impaired production myelin

Metachromatic leukodystrophy

- Three forms
  - Late infantile (6 months to 2 ys)
  - Juvenile (3 to 16 yrs)
  - Adult (age >16)
- Infants/children can present with failure to reach milestones
- Children/adults can have ataxia/dementia

Krabbe's disease

- Lysosomal storage disease
- Autosomal recessive
- Deficiency of galactocerebrosidase
- Buildup of galactocerebroside
- Destroys myelin sheath

Krabbe's disease

- Most patients present <6mo of age
- Progressive motor/sensory problems
- Irritability
- Developmental delay
- Limb spasticity
- Hypotonia
- Absent reflexes
- Microcephaly

Headaches

Jason Ryan, MD, MPH

Headache Causes

- CNS Tumors
- CNS Bleeds (SAH)
- Hydrocephalus
- Inflammation (temporal arteritis)
- In clinical practice, must rule all these things out
- History, exam are key
- Lack of papilledema very important

Primary Headache Disorders

- Tension
- Migraine
- Cluster

Tension Headache

- Very common
- Etiology not clear, probably multifactorial
- Bilateral, constant pain
- Pain is pressing, tightening around head
- 30min to several hours
- Lack of photophobia, phonophobia, or aura
- Diagnosis: clinical
- Treatment: NSAIDs

Migraine Headache

- Unilateral pain
- Pulsating
- Photophobia, phonophobia
- Often nausea, vomiting
- Often has aura
- Clinical diagnosis

Aura

- Gradual development of non-headache symptom
  - Patients will recognize their aura
- About 25% of migraine patients
- Classically precedes HA (but may be same time)
- Often visual
  - Bright, dark spots
  - "Scintillating scotoma"
- Sensory: tingling in limb or face
- Rare auras: speech, motor

Triggers

- Menstruation
- Stress
- Not eating

Migraine Etiology

- Still incompletely understood
- Irritation of CNS structures is important
  - Trigeminal nerve (CNV), meninges, blood vessels
- Activation of trigeminal nerve is important
  - Leads to release of vasoactive neuropeptides
  - Substance P, calcitonin gene-related peptide, neurokinin A
- Sensitization is important
  - Neurons increasingly responsive to stimuli

Migraine Treatment

- Abortive therapy
- Prophylactic Therapy

Abortive Therapy

- Triptans (sumatriptan)
  - 5-HT agonists
  - Inhibit trigeminal nerve
  - ↓vasoactive peptide release
- Also causes vasoconstriction: May raise BP
- Contraindicated:
  - CAD
  - Coronary vasospasm (Prinzmetal's angina)

Abortive Therapy

- Ergotamine
  - Vasoconstrictor
  - Before triptans, major migraine drug
  - Limited by overuse headache, gangrene
- NSAIDs

Preventive Therapy

- Topiramate, Valproate
  - Anticonvulsants
- Propranolol
  - Beta blocker

Topiramate

- Very effective for migraine
- Mental dulling/sedation
- Paresthesias
- Weight LOSS
- Kidney stones
  - Weak carbonic anhydrase inhibitor
  - Leads to more Ca in urine
  - May ↑risk kidney stones
  - Patients need to hydrate

Valproic Acid (Valproate)

- Anti-convulsant
- GI distress, tremor
- Hepatotoxicity (measure LFT's),
- Neural tube defects (spina bifida)
- Weight gain

Propranolol

- Non-selective beta blocker
- Caution:
  - COPD
  - Diabetes
- Fatigue
- Erectile dysfunction

Pregnancy and Migraines

- Usually less headaches while pregnant
- Triptans are okay for abortive
- Avoid: Anti-convulsants, ergotamine, NSAIDs

Cluster Headache

- Very rare
- Poorly understood mechanism
- Mostly men (classic presentation)
- More common in smokers
- Excruciating, unilateral headache behind eye
- Lacrimation, rhinorrhea
- Autonomic dysfunction
  - Horner's syndrome: ptosis, miosis
- Unlike migraine: no aura, no nausea/vomiting

Cluster Headache

- Come in clusters: attacks daily for few weeks
- Circadian rhythm:
  - Daily attacks (same time of day)
- Attacks last 15min to several hours
  - Contrast with trigeminal neuralgia: <1min
- Treatment: Oxygen, triptans
  - Mechanism for oxygen unclear
  - May be related to O2 induced vasoconstriction
  - O2 also inhibits neuronal activation in the trigeminal nucleus

Brain Tumors

Jason Ryan, MD, MPH

Brain Tumors

Adult	Children
· Glioblastoma	· Astrocytoma
· Meningioma	· Medulloblastoma
· Schwannoma	· Ependymoma
· Oligodendroma	· Hemangioblastoma
· Pituitary Adenoma	· Craniopharyngioma

Most adult tumors above tentorium: Supratentorial

Most child tumors below tentorium: Infratentorial

Brain Tumors

- Primary 50%
- Secondary 50%
  - Multiple lesions
  - Most common: Lung, breast, renal

Symptoms

- Headache
- Seizures
- Motor/sensory symptoms

Treatment

- Surgery
- Radiation
- Chemotherapy
- Different depending on type of tumor

Glioblastoma

- Most common primary brain tumor adults
- Occurs in cerebral cortex
- Rapidly progressive, malignant
- Usually fatal <1year
- Half of patients >65
- Older age = worse prognosis
- Often crosses corpus callosum
  - Butterfly glioma
- Express GFAP

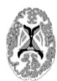

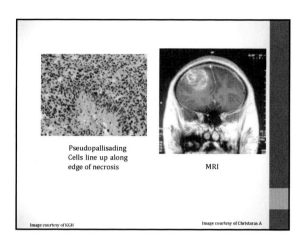

Pseudopallisading
Cells line up along
edge of necrosis

MRI

Image courtesy of KGH

Image courtesy of Christaras A

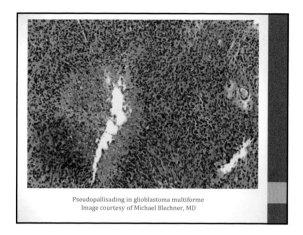

Pseudopallisading in glioblastoma multiforme
Image courtesy of Michael Blechner, MD

Meningioma

- 2nd most common brain tumor
- Convexities of hemispheres near surfaces of brain
- Arise from arachnoid cells
- "Extra-axial" - external to brain
- Can have dural attachment ("tail")

Meningioma

- Usually benign (no mets) and resectable
- Often asymptomatic
- Sometimes seizures
- Classically affects female more than males
  - Expresses estrogen receptors
- Prior radiation to head is risk factor
  - Childhood malignancies
  - Latency period ~20years

Meningioma

Image courtesy of Nephron

Parasagittal Meningioma

- Will compress the leg area similar to ACA stroke
- Classic presentation

Meningioma

Psammoma body

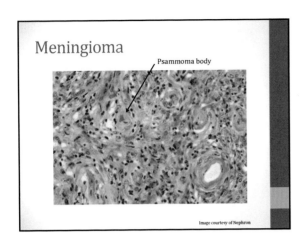

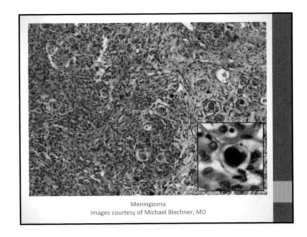

Meningioma
Images courtesy of Michael Blechner, MD

Schwannoma

- 3rd most common adult primary brain tumor
- Schwann cells are glial (non neurons) of PNS
- Classically located to CN VIII
- Hearing loss, tinnitus, ataxia
- Cerebellopontine angle symptoms
  - Facial nerve and vestibulocochlear nerve emerge here
- Treatable with surgery, radiation
- Stain positive for protein S-100

Schwannoma

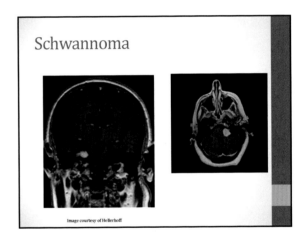

Neurofibromatosis

- Autosomal dominant disease
- Mutation NF1 /NF2 genes
- Neurofibromas
- Lisch nodules
- Café-au-lait spots

Neurofibromatosis

- Type 1:
  - Most common
  - Café-au-lait spots, Neurofibromas
- Type 2:
  - Bilateral schwannomas (almost all patients)
  - Meningiomas
  - Multiple tumors
  - MISME: Multiple inherited schwannomas, meningiomas, and ependymomas

Oligodendroglioma

- Rare tumors
- Slow growing
- Usually in frontal lobe
- Often presents with seizures
- Tumor of white matter

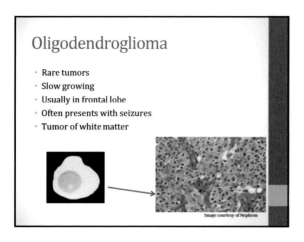

Image courtesy of Nephron

Pituitary adenoma

- Benign (usually) growths of pituitary gland
- Often cause endocrine symptoms
  - Hypo/hyper secretion of hormones
- Most commonly secrete prolactin
  - Amenorrhea, galactorrhea, impotence
- Headache
- Bitemporal hemianopsia
- <10mm = microadenoma
- >10mm = macroadenoma

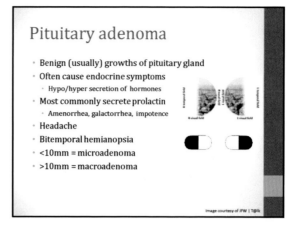

Image courtesy of JFW | T@lk

Pituitary adenoma

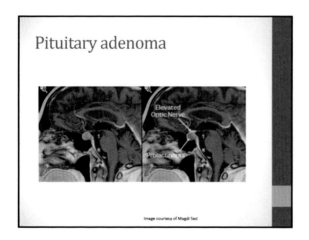

Image courtesy of Magdi Sasi

Childhood CNS Tumors

- Pilocytic astrocytoma ⎤
- Medulloblastoma   ⎬ Cerebellar
- Ependymoma   ⎦
- Craniopharyngioma

Pilocytic astrocytoma

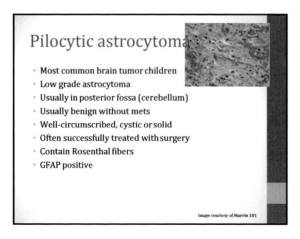

- Most common brain tumor children
- Low grade astrocytoma
- Usually in posterior fossa (cerebellum)
- Usually benign without mets
- Well-circumscribed, cystic or solid
- Often successfully treated with surgery
- Contain Rosenthal fibers
- GFAP positive

Image courtesy of Marvin 101

Medulloblastoma

- Highly malignant primary brain tumor
- Usually occurs in children
- Usually occurs in cerebellum
  - Often in midline (truncal ataxia)
- Type of primitive neuroectodermal tumor (PNET)

Medulloblastoma

- Treatment: Surgery, radiation, chemo
- 75% children survive to adulthood
  - Many with complications of treatment
- Can compress 4th ventricle → hydrocephalus
- Can spread to CSF
  - Nodules in dura of spinal cord: "Drop metastasis"
  - Tend to occur in lower spinal cord, cauda equina
  - Back pain, focal neuro lesions can occur

Medulloblastoma

- Homer-Wrights Rosettes

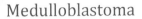

Image courtesy of Eusebius   Image courtesy of Jensflorian

Ependymoma

- Ependyma: epithelium-like lining of ventricles
- Found in brain and the spinal cord
- Often found in 4th ventricle
- Can cause hydrocephalus

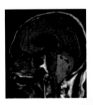

Image courtesy of Hellerhoff

Pseudorosette

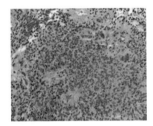

Cells surrounding central core but core is blood vessel

Image courtesy of Nephron

Pseudorosette

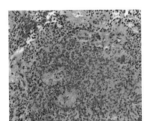

Cells surrounding central core but core is blood vessel

Image courtesy of Nephron

Hemangioblastoma

- Very rare, slow growing CNS tumors
- Often cerebellar, also brainstem & spinal cord
- Well-circumscribed, highly vascular

Hemangioblastoma

- Two key facts to know
- #1: Can produce EPO → polycythemia (↑Hct)
- #2: Occur in von Hippel-Lindau syndrome
  - Autosomal dominant disease
  - Tumor suppressor gene mutation
  - LOTS of tumors
  - Hemangioblastomas of the brain (cerebellum) and spine
  - Retinal angiomas
  - Renal cell carcinomas (RCCs)
  - Pheochromocytomas

Craniopharyngioma

- Mostly children 10-14 years old
  - Rarely younger adults
- Suprasellar
  - Anywhere pituitary gland → base 3rd ventricle
- Benign
- Symptoms from compression
  - Visual field defects
  - Hormonal imbalance
  - Behavioral change (frontal lobe dysfunction)

Craniopharyngioma

- Derived from remnants of Rathke's pouch
  - Invagination of the ectoderm
  - Protrudes from roof of mouth
  - Also forms anterior pituitary
- Often calcified and cystic
- Contain epithelial cells
  - Appearances similar to pulp of developing teeth
- Can compress optic chiasm
  - Bitemporal hemianopsia

Craniopharyngioma

Image courtesy of Dr.Roopchand.PS

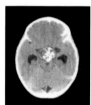

Image courtesy of Matthew R Garnett

Pineal Tumors

- Rare germ cell tumors or parenchymal tumors
- Compression pretectal area of midbrain
- Parinaud syndrome
  - Paralysis of upward gaze
  - Pseudo-Argyll-Robertson pupils
  - React to accommodation but not light
- Can compress cerebral aqueduct
  - Hydrocephalus, papilledema

Parkinson's, Huntington's, and Movement Disorders

Jason Ryan, MD, MPH

Movement Disorders

- Parkinson's disease
- Huntington's Disease

- Wilson's Disease
- All result from damage to part of basal ganglia

Basal Ganglia Connections

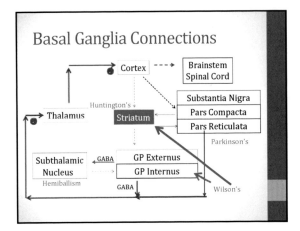

Cortex - - - → Brainstem / Spinal Cord

Substantia Nigra
Pars Compacta
Pars Reticulata

Huntington's
Thalamus → Striatum
Parkinson's

Subthalamic Nucleus ← GABA → GP Externus
GP Internus
Hemiballism
GABA
Wilson's

Parkinson's Disease

- Degenerative disease of substantia nigra
- Depletion of dopamine in SN Pars Compacta
- Loss of melanin-containing dopaminergic neurons SN
  - Depigmentation
- Pathologic hallmark: Lewy bodies in SN
  - Inclusion in neurons of α-synuclein

Image courtesy of Charles E. Driscoll, MD

MPTP

- Methyl-phenyl-tetrahydropyridine
- Destroys dopamine neurons
- Causes Parkinson's
- May be contaminant of opioid drugs

Parkinson's Disease

- Classic case: older, male patient
  - Average age onset in 60s
- Rest tremor (pill-rolling tremor)
- Bradykinesia – can't initiate movements
- Movement gets better with exercise
- Shuffling gate
- Stooped posture
- Cogwheel rigidity

Parkinson's Treatments

Drug	Mechanism
L-dopa/carbidopa	Converted to dopamine in CNS
Entacapone, Tolcapone	COMT inhibitors; prevent L-dopa breakdown
Selegiline	Prevents dopamine breakdown
Bromocriptine	Dopamine agonist (ergot)
Pramipexole, Ropinirole	Dopamine agonists (non-ergot)
Benztropine, Trihexyphenidyl	Antimuscarinic
Propranolol	Beta blocker
Amantadine	Dopamine agonists, anticholinergic (also an antiviral)

L-dopa/carbidopa
Sinemet

- L-dopa crosses blood-brain barrier
- Converted to dopamine in CNS
  - Dopa decarboxylase
- Peripheral decarboxylase can breakdown L-dopa
  - This limits its benefit
  - Also creates peripheral dopa
  - Can cause heart side effects
  - Can cause nausea/vomiting (vomiting center outside BBB)

L-dopa/carbidopa
Sinemet

- Carbidopa inhibits peripheral decarboxylase
- Given together: L-dopa/Carbidopa
- Still get CNS side effects of L-dopa
  - L-dopa becomes dopa in CNS
  - Anxiety, agitation, insomnia
- Use lowest dose possible
- Avoid vitamin B6

L-dopa/carbidopa
Sinemet

- Long-term use → Motor side effects
- Drug reduces natural L-dopa production
- "On-off" phenomenon
- Akinesia occurs between doses
- Involuntary movements
- Use lowest dose possible to avoid

Entacapone and Tolcapone

- Inhibit catechol-O-methyltransferase (COMT)
- Enzyme that breaks down L-dopa
  - Even with carbidopa, COMT limits L-dopa benefit
- Only work in combination with L-dopa
- Entacapone: peripheral COMT inhibition
- Tolcapone: peripheral and central COMT inhibition
- Tolcapone associated with hepatotoxicity

Selegiline

- Inhibits MAO-b
  - Central dopamine breakdown enzyme
  - Breaks down dopamine more than 5HT
- Increases central dopamine levels
- Can be added to L-dopa/carbidopa
- Side effects:
  - Nausea, vomiting
  - Hypotension
  - Excessive daytime sleepiness

Selegiline
Side Effects

- Serotonin syndrome
  - When given with SSRI
  - Confusion, fever, myoclonus
- "Cheese effect"
  - Hypertensive crisis
  - Tyramine foods: Red wine, aged cheese, or aged meat
  - MAO inhibitors (a or b) block breakdown of tyramine
  - Tyramine → HTN

Parkinson's Drugs

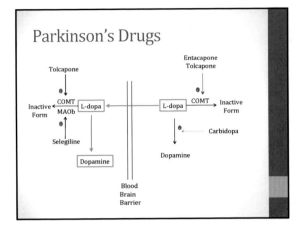

Parkinson Drugs in Practice

- Tremor predominant symptoms
  - Trihexyphenidyl (anti-muscarinic)
  - Side effects: sedation, dry mouth
- Bradykinesia, rigidity
  - Ropinirole, pramipexole (dopamine agonists)
  - Levodopa/carbidopa

Surgical Therapy Parkinson's

- Young patients often develop toxicity from long term use of L-dopa/carbidopa
- Prior surgeries used:
  - Pallidotomy (partial ablation of globus pallidus)
  - Thalamotomy (partial ablation of thalamus)
- Modern option: Deep brain stimulation
  - High frequency DBS suppresses neural activation

Huntington's Disease

- Inherited autosomal dominant disorder
- Degeneration in striatum
  - Striatum = caudate + putamen
  - Loss of GABA neurons (also ACh)
- Brain imaging
  - Lateral ventricles may appear large
  - Marked caudate degeneration
- Also has atrophy of frontal/temporal lobes

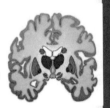

Huntington's Disease

- Mutation in the HTT gene
- CAG repeat in gene
- Normal 10-35 repeats
- Huntington's 36 to 120 repeats
- Worse/earlier symptoms each generation
  - "Anticipation"
- Neuronal death from glutamate toxicity
  - Glutamate binds NMDA receptor
  - Excessive influx calcium
  - Cell death

Huntington's Disease

- Onset of symptoms 30s-40s
- Death after 10-20 years
- Chorea
- Aggression
- Depression
- Dementia
- Can be mistaken for substance abuse

Huntington's Treatment

- Dopamine associated with chorea
- Blocking dopamine can reduce chorea
- Tetrabenazine and reserpine
  - Inhibit VMAT
  - Limit dopamine vesicle packaging /release
- Haloperidol
  - Dopamine receptor antagonist

Hemibalism

- Wild, flinging movements of extremities (ballistic)
- Damage to subthalamic nuclues
- Seen in rare subtypes of lacunar strokes

Wilson's Disease

- Disorder of Copper metabolism
- Leads to accumulation of copper in tissues
- Lesions occur in basal ganglia
  - Lentiform nucleus (putamen/globus pallidus)
- Movement symptoms
  - Can be parkinsonian
  - Wing-beating tremor
  - Dysarthria

Other movement disorders

Disorder	Appearance	Lesion
Chorea	Random, purposeless movements	Basal ganglia
Athetosis	Slow, writhing movements of fingers	Basal ganglia
Myoclonus	Sudden muscle contraction, jerk, twitch	Can occur renal/liver failure
Dystonia	Sudden contractions; twitching	Writer's cramp; blepharospasm

Chorea

- Two important causes:
  - Huntington's disease
  - Acute rheumatic fever
- History is key

Tremors

Type	Appearance	Comments
Essential Tremor	Occurs with intentional movement	--
Resting Tremor	At rest; usually hands; better with intentional movements "pill rolling"	Classic for Parkinson's
Intention Tremor	Zig-zag motion when trying to move finger toward target	Cerebellar dysfunction; "Finger to nose" test
Wing-beating Tremor	Hands clasped together, elbows out, flapping	Wilson's disease

Essential Tremor

- Old name: "Benign familial tremor"
  - Distinguish from Parkinson's
- Genetic predisposition
- EtOH helps – patients self-medicate
- Drug treatment
  - Propranolol (beta blocker)
  - Primidone

HIV CNS Infections

Jason Ryan, MD, MPH

CNS Infections in HIV Patients

- Cryptococcus
- Cytomegalovirus (CMV)
- Toxoplasmosis
- JC virus
  - Progressive multifocal leukoencephalopathy (PML)

Cryptococcus Neoformans

- Invasive fungus
- Thick polysaccharide capsule
- Present in soil and pigeon droppings

Cryptococcus Neoformans

- Inhaled → lungs → blood stream → meninges
- Can also occur immunocompromised
  - Chemo, post-transplant

Cryptococcus Neoformans

- Indolent symptoms over weeks
  - Fever, headache
- Can cause ↑ICP
- Risk of herniation with LP
- Must do CT or MRI
- Treatment: Amphotericin B or Fluconazole

Cryptococcus Neoformans

- Sabouraud's agar
- Latex agglutination test
  - Detects polysaccharide capsular antigen
- Soap bubble lesions on MRI

Cryptococcus Neoformans

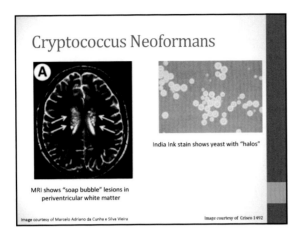

India Ink stain shows yeast with "halos"

MRI shows "soap bubble" lesions in periventricular white matter

Image courtesy of Marcelo Adriano da Cunha e Silva Vieira   Image courtesy of Crisco 1492

CMV Retinitis

- Retinal edema/necrosis
- Floaters, ↓vision
- CMV in HIV/AIDS:
  - Low CD4 (50-100)

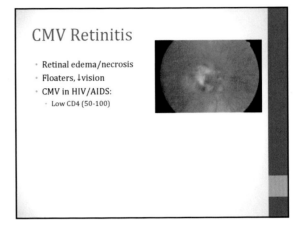

Toxoplasma gondii

- Multiple "ring-enhancing" lesions on imaging
- CD4 <100cells/mm3
- Treatment: Sulfadiazine/pyrimethamine

Image courtesy of LearningRadiology.com

Progressive multifocal leukoencephalopathy (PML)

- Severe demyelinating disease of CNS
- Reactivation of a latent JC virus → demyelination
- CD4 < 200 cells/mm3
- Causes slow onset encephalopathy
  - Altered mental status
  - Focal neuro defects (motor, gait, etc)
- Dx: JC Virus DNA in CSF or brain biopsy

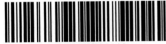
Made in the USA
Lexington, KY
07 November 2018